Life Support

Anthony J Handley MD FRCP

Technical Contributors: Olive Bowes and David Eaton

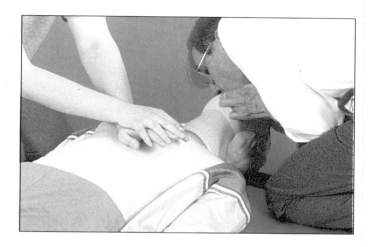

Contents in Brief

Introduction 2

Life Support 10

Techniques 16

Lifesaving First Aid 40

Drowning, Hypothermia and Life Support 52

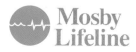 Mosby
Lifeline

St. Louis Baltimore Carlsbad Philadelphia
London Sydney Tokyo Toronto

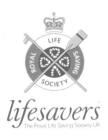

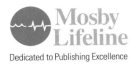

Dedicated to Publishing Excellence

Life Support

Anthony J Handley MD FRCP
Chief Medical Advisor, RLSS UK

Technical Contributors: **Olive Bowes and David Eaton**

Publisher: John A Hirst
Vice President, Publishing Technology: Adam Phillips
Sales and Marketing Director: Christy J Wilson
Production Director: Susan Walby
Production Controller: Gudrun Hughes
Book Design: Studio Montage
Location Photography: Tim Fisher, Lila Bahl
Studio Photography: Medical Photographic Department, Essex Rivers Healthcare NHS Trust

Author's note
Throughout my text the masculine includes the feminine
(unless the context dictates otherwise), and vice versa.

Acknowledgements

RLSS UK would like to thank:

RLSS UK National Lifesaving Committee and volunteers; River House staff; Essex Rivers Healthcare NHS Trust; Kab Pressings, Studley; The Leys Sports Centre, Redditch; John Hirst, Christy Wilson and Fiona Alderman at Mosby Lifeline; Studio Montage; residents of Broadwell and Sedgeberrow; Tim Fisher and Lila Bahl.

Real life examples

The stories illustrating life support action all portray real incidents. Generally, the names and locations have been changed to protect the privacy of the individuals concerned. Similarly, most of the photographs were posed by models rather than the people involved.

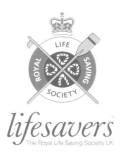

The Royal Life Saving Society UK
River House
Broom
Warwickshire B50 4HN.
Telephone: 01789 773994 Fax: 01789 773995
email: lifesavers@rlss.org.uk

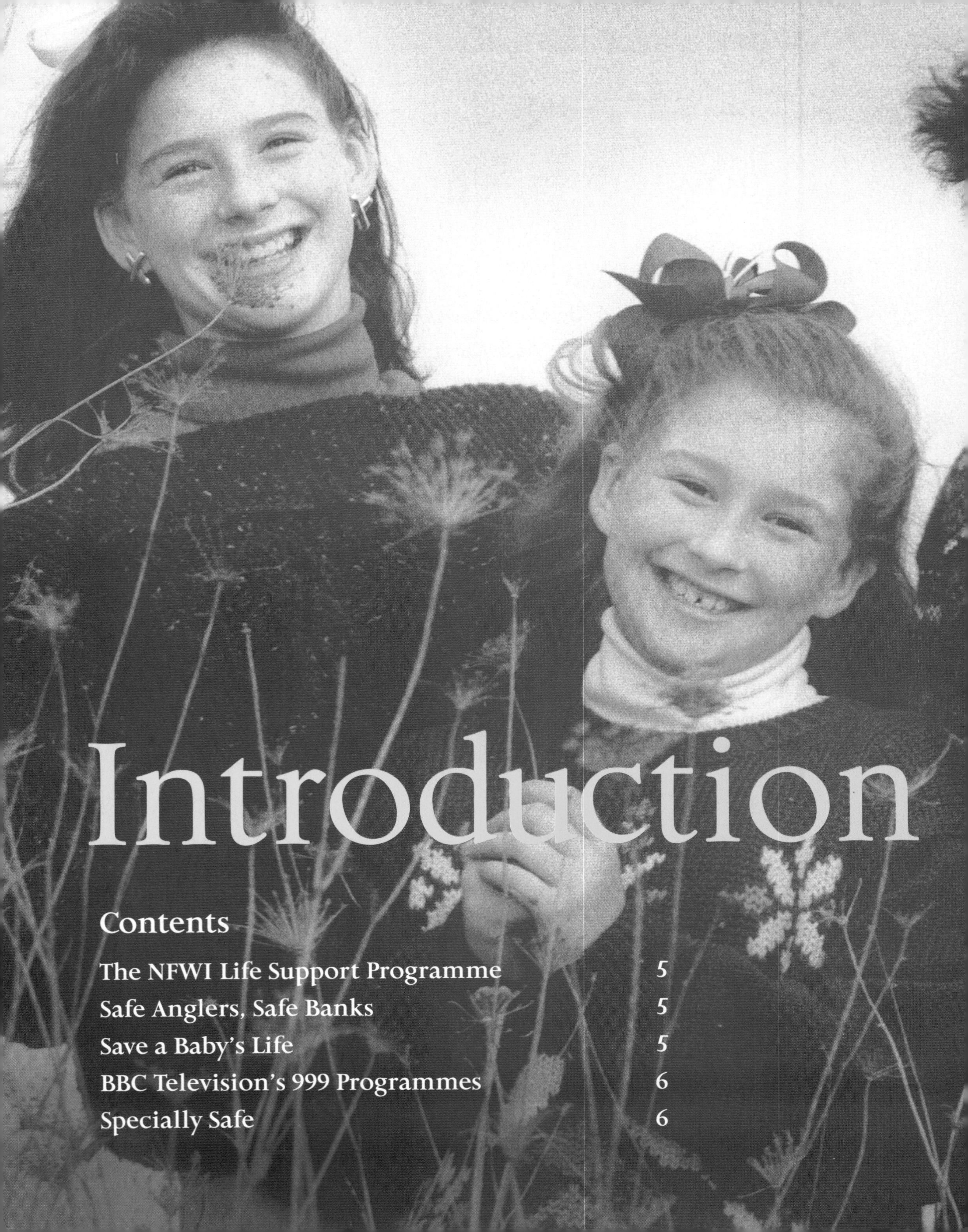

Introduction

Contents

The NFWI Life Support Programme 5

Safe Anglers, Safe Banks 5

Save a Baby's Life 5

BBC Television's 999 Programmes 6

Specially Safe 6

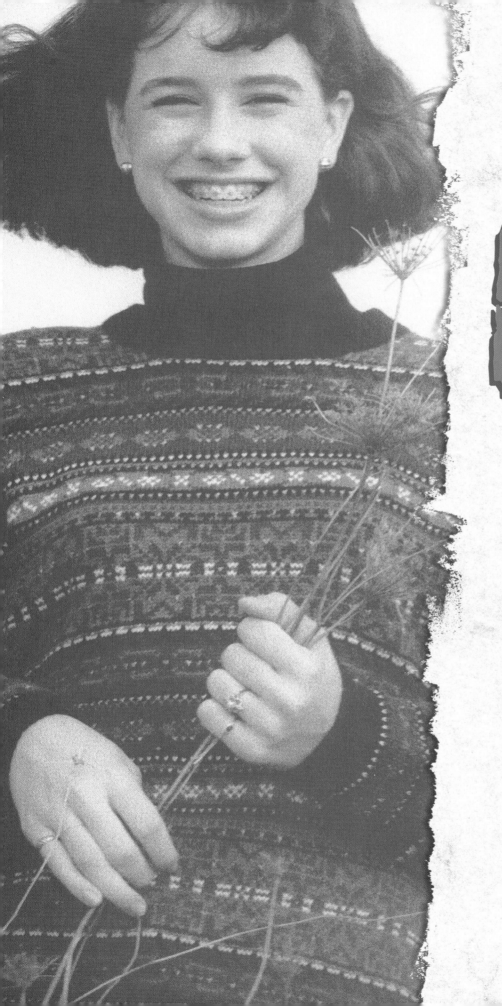

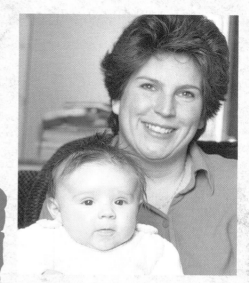

It was every parents' worst nightmare. Darren and Louise Wilson were watching television when Louise thought she heard an unfamiliar sound from the baby intercom. Hurrying upstairs, she found their 3-month-old son Oliver lying still in his cot. "His face was blue." Louise recalled. "I can't describe the terror I felt, how I had to overcome a wave of sheer panic."

Louise fought to remember the life support advice she had received at the clinic as part of the Save a Baby's Life campaign. Calling to Darren to summon an ambulance, she gave Oliver rescue breaths just as the instructor had shown her. By the time she heard the siren, her son was breathing again.

If only I'd known what to do!

*t*raining in basic life support saves lives. Resuscitation and lifesaving first aid immediately after an emergency — an accident, a heart attack or a near-drowning — is crucial. By the time qualified medical aid arrives, it may be too late.

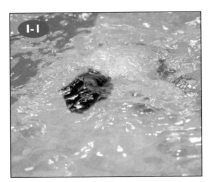

But could YOU save someone's life in an emergency? Would you know what to do if your elderly father suffered a heart attack? ...or if your baby stopped breathing? ...or if you found your partner or child floating unconscious (Figure I-1)? A knowledge of basic life support could literally mean the difference between life and death to your loved ones, friends, neighbours and fellow citizens (Figure I-2).

Each year, thousands of needless deaths could be prevented if there was someone on hand who had been trained to carry out rescue breathing (the 'kiss of life') and keep blood circulating by applying chest compressions.

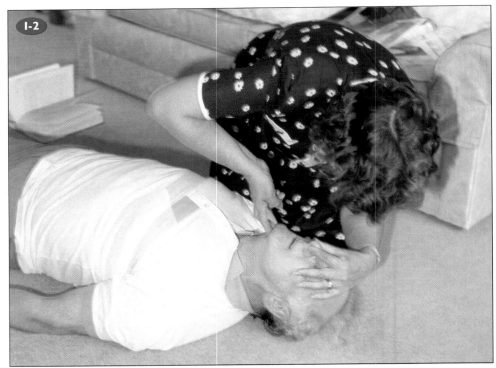

The combination of these two techniques (called cardiopulmonary resuscitation) can support life until a doctor or ambulance arrives.

The more members of the public who are trained in resuscitation and lifesaving first aid, the more lives can be saved. The Royal Life Saving Society, the longest-established water safety charity in the world, is the UK's leading authoritative source of lifesaving training and education.

Since RLSS was founded in 1891, the number of people who drown in Britain has fallen steadily year after year. Today, the figure is little over one tenth of what it was a century ago. Life support training is an essential element of our world-renowned awards scheme – the Bronze Medallion, the Award of Merit and the Distinction – and of our National Lifeguard Qualification programmes. Life support skills for children form an important part of our popular and successful Rookie Lifesaver Training Programme (Figure I-3). Following the successful Swim For Life Campaign, life support is an option in the swimming activity at Key Stages 3 and 4 of the National Curriculum in England and Wales.

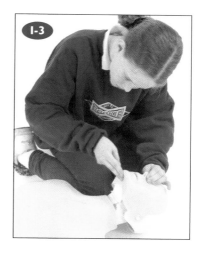

Despite our success in drowning prevention and water rescue, thousands more lives could be saved each year if every citizen knew how to give life support in other emergency situations. That is why we continue to promote and develop lifesaving techniques and cascade these skills into the community through our network of highly qualified trainers. Reaching out to the community is a vital part of our work.

Some of our highly effective outreach programmes are described on page 5. They are targeted at vulnerable sections of society such as infants or highly stressed middle-aged men where immediate life support is so often a matter of life or death. We are constantly looking for new ways to reach the community with programmes designed to attract the widest range of common interests and activities.

Jim Mills had just retired when he had his heart attack. His wife, Rosemary, heard the crash as he fell from his chair grasping his chest. By the time she reached the sitting room, Jim was no longer breathing. Luckily, Rosemary knew what to do, having just completed a life support training course with her local Women's Institute. She grabbed the telephone and dialled.

Once the ambulance was on its way, she cleared Jim's airway and started rescue breathing as she had been shown. When her husband failed to respond, Rosemary began chest compressions. Her prompt action bought precious time until the paramedics arrived with their advanced life support equipment.

"Rosie never thought she'd have to put her course into practice so soon... but without that training I'd have been gone."

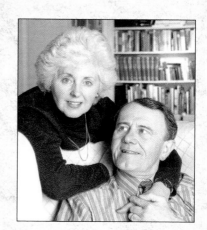

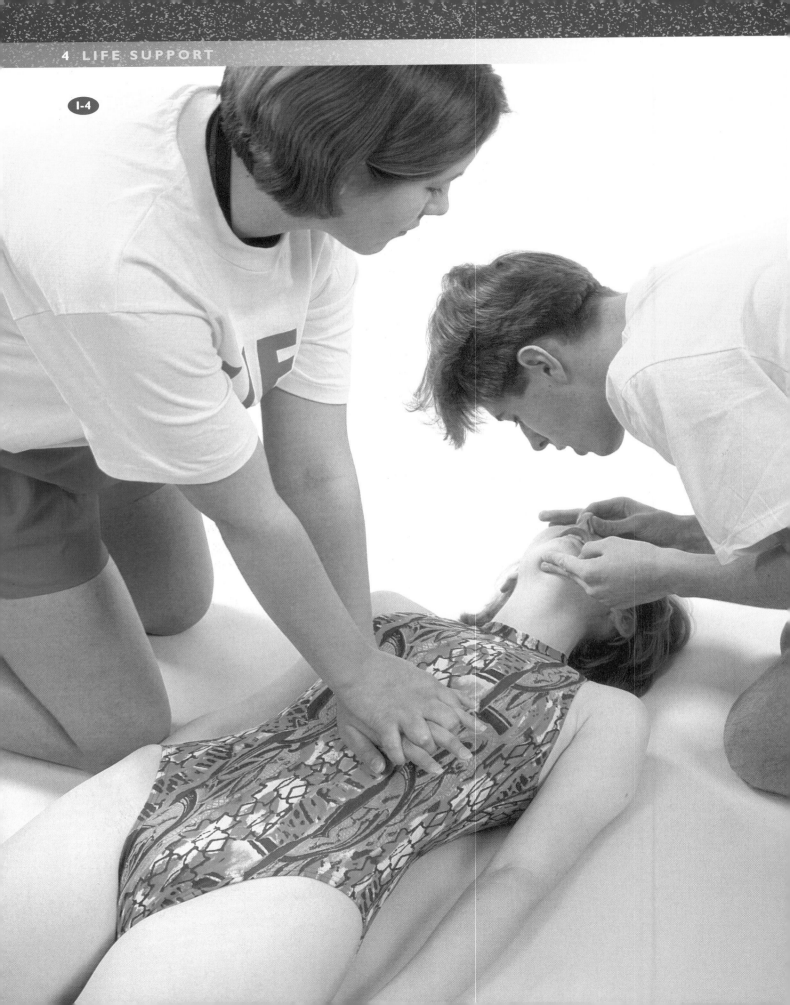

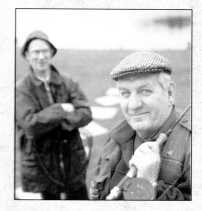

As well as our water-related activities, RLSS UK's current major campaigns include:

The NFWI Life Support Programme

This programme is a partnership between RLSS UK and the National Federation of Women's Institutes. Nearly two thirds of all victims of fatal cardiac arrest are men in their homes. So it is vital that the person most likely to be around when a heart attack strikes — the victim's partner — has received life support training. The programme is designed to bring basic life support skills to the 250,000 (latest NFWI count) members of 8,000 Women's Institutes throughout Britain.

Safe Anglers, Safe Banks

Over two million anglers enjoy their sport beside Britain's lakes, rivers, reservoirs, canals and coastline. An angler is likely to be the first on the scene in over half of all drownings and water emergencies. Our *Safe Anglers, Safe Banks* programme is designed to equip anglers with the skills to make them highly effective lifesavers. Another benefit is that the water safety skills element of the programme will reduce the number of anglers who drown each year (Figure I-5).

Save a Baby's Life

A baby is particularly vulnerable during the crucial first months of its life. This is also a very worrying period for first time mums and dads who, through inexperience, may not know what to do if an emergency arises.

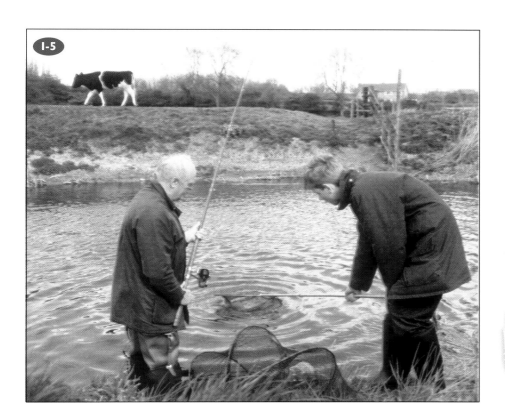

I-5

A quiet day's angling turned into a drama for Alf Barrett. The retired postman was alarmed to see a hand projecting from the water and below it the dark silhouette of a man.

Alf waded into the shallow water and hauled the angler to the bank. The man seemed lifeless with no pulse or signs of breathing. "My local club runs Safe Anglers, Safe Banks training sessions," says Alf, "so I knew what to do. I called the emergency services on my mobile phone then gave cardiopulmonary resuscitation."

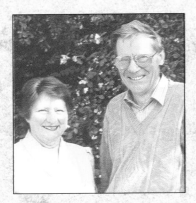

G wen organises life support courses for the joint RLSS UK and National Federation of Women's Institute life support training project. Two weeks after she attended an instructors' course run by RLSS UK's Suffolk Branch, her husband Ted became ill one evening. Gwen put her knowledge to good use and Ted was rushed to hospital.

Within a month, Gwen's lifesaving skill helped her husband survive two more cardiac arrests.

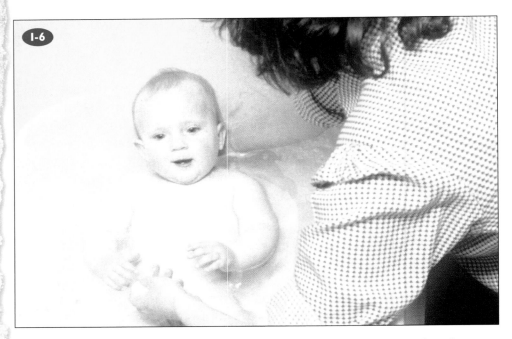

I-6

The *Save a Baby's Life* programme, in partnership with ante-natal and post-natal healthcare professionals, will provide life support training to those who care for babies. It will give them the skills to deal with emergencies such as choking on food, smothering by pets or bedclothes, near-drownings at bath-time (Figure I-6), or cot death.

BBC Television's 999 Programmes

RLSS UK's lifesaving expertise provides a valuable resource for the popular BBC Television programmes *999* and *999 Lifesaver*. We have been a major partner in the BBC's *999 Lifesaver Roadshows*. At these events, staged throughout the UK, members of the public learn basic lifesaving and life support skills from highly skilled trainers (Figure 1-7). Already, the roadshows have equipped over 10,000 people with the skills to save lives.

Specially Safe

This RLSS UK training programme helps people with disabilities enjoy swimming safely. *Specially Safe* offers complete guidance to anyone supervising or organising swimming activities for them. With support from The Foundation for Sport and The Arts, the programme includes a training manual, a video cassette and a supporting award programme, the *Rescue Test for Supervisors of Swimmers with Disabilities*.

Training in life support, resuscitation, and lifesaving first aid are at the heart of all these programmes and the purpose of this book is to support and develop that training. It is not aimed at medical professionals (although they will find much of value in the following pages) but at anyone who wants to know how to save a life in an emergency. It will also be of particular value to people who wish to teach lifesaving skills through the community outreach programmes described above or as part of RLSS UK's awards or qualifications.

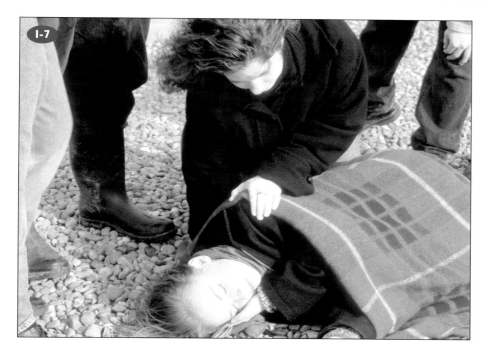

Learning the skills in this book will enable you to respond in the right way if an emergency occurs. Once learned, your skills must be practised and kept up to date. Research shows that without this continuing interest and involvement, you may forget half your lifesaving skills after as little as six months. Rather than finding this discouraging, it spurs us on to develop interesting and stimulating ways to ensure that, once you have mastered the techniques of life support, you will want to develop and practise your skills regularly.

Above all, we know that after proper training your actions in an emergency will always be more effective than doing nothing.

Finally, if you would like to help us bring the gift of lifesaving training to as many people as possible, please turn to the back of this book where you will find a tear-out card which tells you how you can support our work. We can't save lives without YOU.

Stephen Lear
Director, RLSS UK

1

Life Support

Contents

Priorities   11
Control   11
Safety   11
Assessment   11
Life Support Actions   12
Choking   12
Bleeding   12
Unconscious Breathing Casualties   12
Shock   12
Medical Attention   13

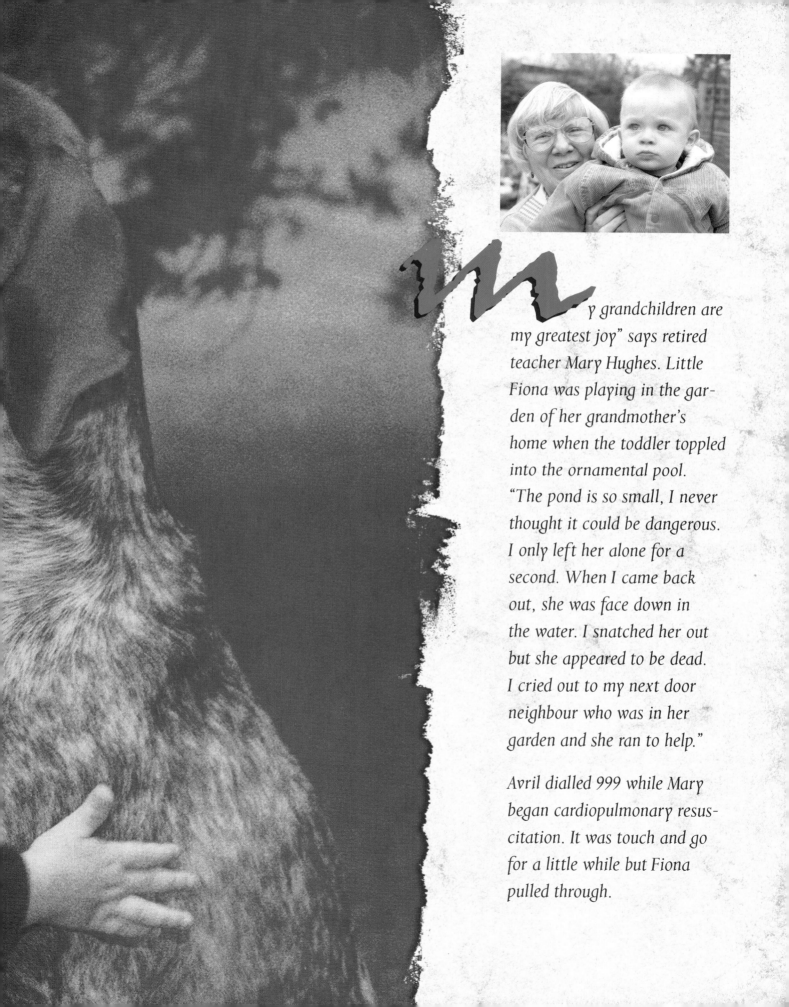

y grandchildren are my greatest joy" says retired teacher Mary Hughes. Little Fiona was playing in the garden of her grandmother's home when the toddler toppled into the ornamental pool. "The pond is so small, I never thought it could be dangerous. I only left her alone for a second. When I came back out, she was face down in the water. I snatched her out but she appeared to be dead. I cried out to my next door neighbour who was in her garden and she ran to help."

Avril dialled 999 while Mary began cardiopulmonary resuscitation. It was touch and go for a little while but Fiona pulled through.

Life Support

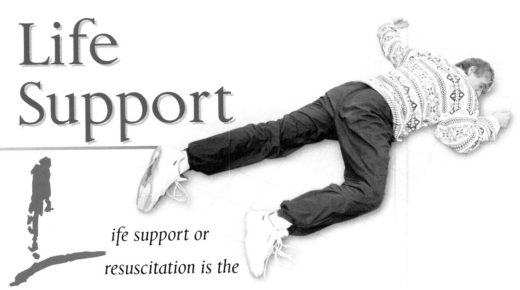

ife support or resuscitation is the emergency help given to a casualty whose heart has stopped (cardiac arrest) or who has stopped breathing.

From the moment of reaching a casualty until he or she can be transferred to the care of more skilled or qualified personnel, individual lifesavers will be responsible for resuscitation and any other lifesaving first aid required. Although speed and decisiveness are essential, care must be taken that hasty measures do not worsen the condition of the casualty or endanger the rescuers.

The aims of life support and lifesaving first aid are:

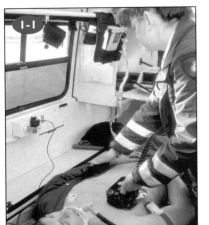

- to preserve life; and
- to obtain further qualified assistance without delay (Figure 1-1).

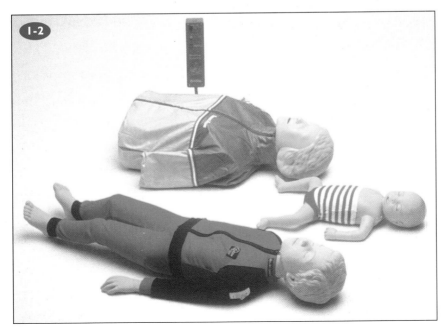

To be able to achieve these aims life-savers must be well trained (Figure 1-2) and able to assume responsibility for managing casualties. Through tuition from medically qualified or lay teachers, lifesavers should obtain recognized qualifications such as the resuscitation awards of the Royal Life Saving Society UK and the first aid certificates of St John Ambulance, St Andrew's Ambulance Association or the British Red Cross Society. Thereafter, they should keep up-to-date and improve their basic knowledge and skills.

Priorities

When attending any emergency or incident, the would-be rescuer should undertake the following as necessary:

- control;
- safety;
- assessment; and
- lifesaving actions.

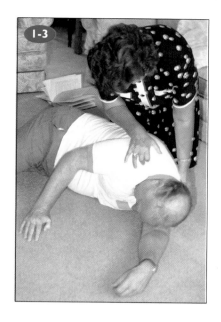

Control

On arriving at the scene of the emergency, state that you are a trained lifesaver. If there are no doctors, nurses or medically more experienced people present, take charge calmly but firmly.

Spend a few moments collecting your thoughts, assessing the need for safety precautions and gaining an overall impression of the nature of the emergency with which you have to cope (Figure 1-3).

Safety

Minimize as far as possible the risk of any further harm coming to the casualty, bearing in mind the need for your own safety and that of other rescuers. Where possible remove danger from the casualty, rather than the casualty from danger, for example by controlling road traffic. Occasionally it may be necessary to move the casualty before even the most urgent resuscitation is carried out. For instance, the casualty might be in a gas-filled room.

Assessment

The way you plan your assistance will depend on the number of able-bodied helpers you have available. You may be able to include those who have been involved in the incident once they have been rescued and provided they are not seriously injured or suffering from shock. Determine quickly the capability and training of any potential helpers. Have they been taught first aid or resuscitation? Do they know the procedure for calling an ambulance?

When more than one casualty is involved in an incident it is important to treat the most seriously affected first. When dealing with an individual casualty, life-threatening conditions must be attended to before less serious injuries, and generally in the order below:

- life support;
- management of choking;
- control of life-threatening bleeding;
- care of the unconscious breathing casualty; and
- treatment for shock.

It is important to note that sometimes bleeding may be so severe that it must be stopped before resuscitation can be effective.

A description of the management of these conditions follows.

Hopefully, you will rarely have to put your life support knowledge to use. Because of this, your life-saving skills may deteriorate after as little as six months. So it is important to keep in practice and to attend regular refresher courses.

1-4 Life Support

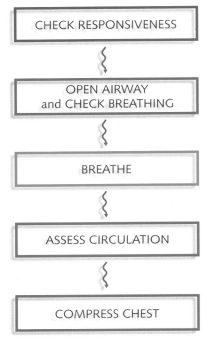

Life Support Actions

Life support actions (chest compression and/or rescue breathing) normally take absolute priority over any other First Aid measures. Details of the techniques are fully described in the next chapter.

In summary, they are as shown in chart (Figure 1-4) on the left.

Choking

Choking occurs when a piece of food or other material is swallowed but goes down the trachea (windpipe) rather than the oesophagus (gullet). This results in blockage of the airway. If this blockage is only partial the casualty will usually be able to dislodge it by coughing, but if there is complete obstruction to flow of air, this may not be possible. Unless help is given urgently the casualty will suffer from suffocation, become unconscious and may die. Even a small piece of food such as a peanut may cause serious obstruction because its presence can lead to muscle spasm in the region of the larynx (voice box).

You will find more detailed information on how to manage choking in Chapter 3.

Bleeding

If blood is lost, the amount of oxygen that can be carried to the organs and tissues of the body is reduced. If bleeding is severe it can lead to shock and ultimately to death. Bleeding may occur externally (e.g. a cut or graze) or internally (e.g. rupture of the spleen after a blow to the abdomen; bleeding into a muscle after a crush injury). External bleeding is usually obvious but a quick examination of the whole casualty, including any necessary removal of clothing, will ensure that no hidden bleeding is missed. Internal bleeding is difficult to diagnose; signs of shock will occur and the casualty should be treated for this condition.

You will find more detailed information on how to manage bleeding in Chapter 3.

Unconscious Breathing Casualties

Loss of consciousness may occur for a number of different reasons, but whatever the cause, emergency care is basically the same.

You will find more detailed information on how to manage unconscious casualties in Chapter 3.

Shock

Shock can be defined as 'failure of the circulation which results in an inadequate supply of blood to vital organs.' It occurs when, for a number of reasons, there is not enough blood being pumped round the body. Since one of the main functions of blood is to carry oxygen, failure of the circulation means that essential parts of the body such as the brain, kidneys, and heart do not receive as much oxygen as they need and can no longer function properly. Unless the casualty is treated quickly and adequately death may result.

You will find more detailed information on how to manage shock in Chapter 3.

Medical Attention

Unless the injury or incident has been of a very mild nature, medical assistance must be obtained from a doctor or hospital. When in doubt seek advice. Always obtain a medical opinion if:

- the casualty has been unconscious;
- any resuscitation measures have been necessary;
- there are any signs of shock; or
- the casualty has been totally submerged under water (Figure 1-5).

These rules apply even if the casualty appears to have recovered fully.

In the case of a seriously injured or unconscious casualty

After completing first aid measures, you should obtain medical assistance by calling an ambulance. Dial 999 (or 112) from a telephone. Be ready to give the telephone number from which you are calling, brief details of the incident, the location, the number of casualties, the nature of the injuries, the urgency with which an ambulance is required and your own name.

In the case of a mildly injured casualty (or where doubt exists)

After completing first aid measures, you should obtain medical assistance by contacting the nearest General Practitioner or taking the casualty to a doctor's surgery or hospital accident and emergency department.

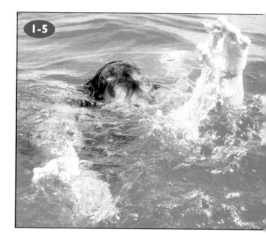

1-5

Chapter One — Test Yourself

1. What is Life Support?

2. What are the aims of Life Support and Lifesaving First Aid?

3. What are the priorities for a rescuer at an emergency?

4. If more than one casualty is involved, how do you decide which to deal with first?

5. What is meant by choking?

6. What is the difference between internal and external bleeding?

7. What is shock?

8. Give four examples of when you should seek medical assistance for a casualty.

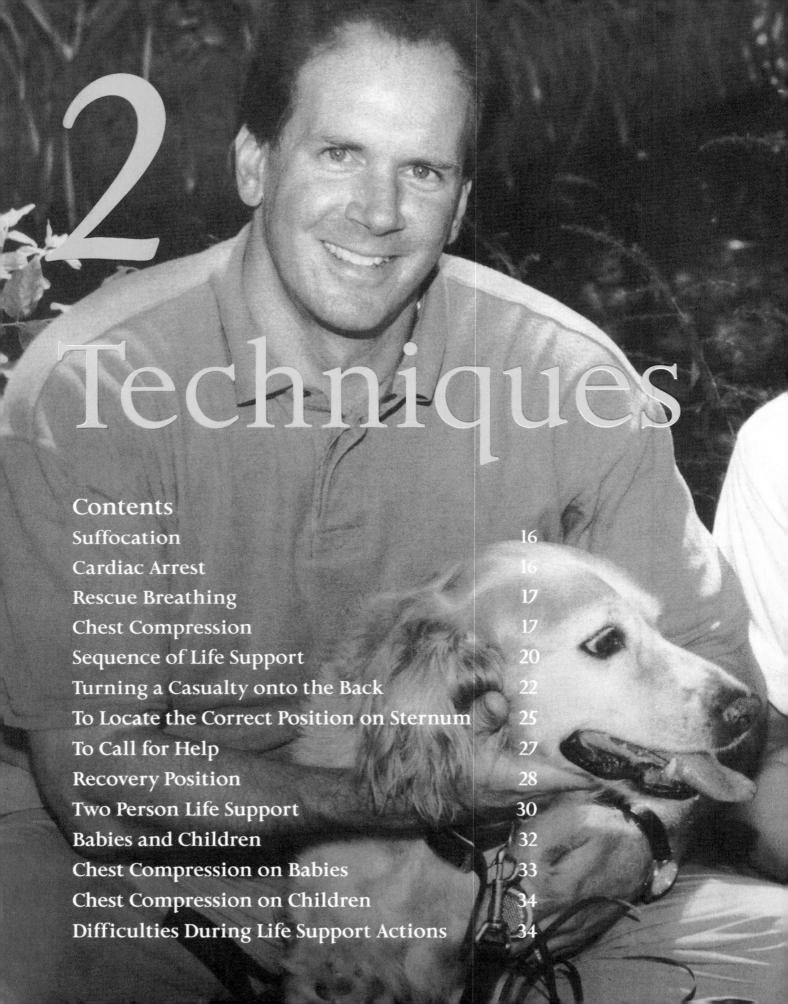

2

Techniques

Contents

Suffocation	16
Cardiac Arrest	16
Rescue Breathing	17
Chest Compression	17
Sequence of Life Support	20
Turning a Casualty onto the Back	22
To Locate the Correct Position on Sternum	25
To Call for Help	27
Recovery Position	28
Two Person Life Support	30
Babies and Children	32
Chest Compression on Babies	33
Chest Compression on Children	34
Difficulties During Life Support Actions	34

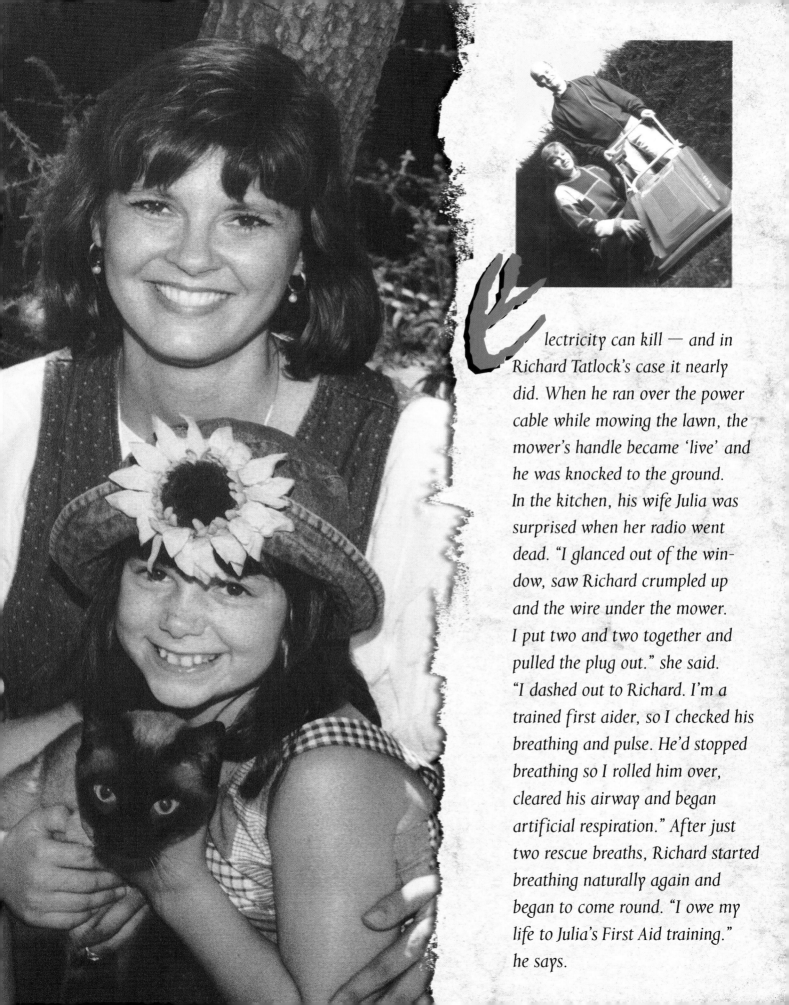

lectricity can kill — and in Richard Tatlock's case it nearly did. When he ran over the power cable while mowing the lawn, the mower's handle became 'live' and he was knocked to the ground. In the kitchen, his wife Julia was surprised when her radio went dead. "I glanced out of the window, saw Richard crumpled up and the wire under the mower. I put two and two together and pulled the plug out." she said. "I dashed out to Richard. I'm a trained first aider, so I checked his breathing and pulse. He'd stopped breathing so I rolled him over, cleared his airway and began artificial respiration." After just two rescue breaths, Richard started breathing naturally again and began to come round. "I owe my life to Julia's First Aid training." he says.

Techniques

I f a casualty's breathing is inadequate (suffocation) or the heart has stopped beating (cardiac arrest), life support action is needed urgently.

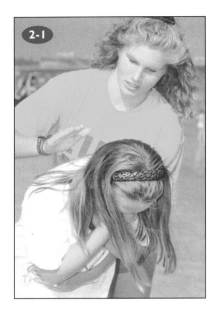

Suffocation

This is the term used to describe any condition in which insufficient air is reaching the lungs to supply the body's need for oxygen. It may be due, for example, to:

- the tongue falling back and blocking the throat in an unconscious casualty;
- a foreign body stuck in the throat (Figure 2-1);
- strangulation; or
- drowning.

Cardiac Arrest

This is the term used to describe the condition in which the heart is no longer pumping blood round the body. The heart may stop beating either because its muscle is not contracting at all (asystole) or because it is twitching in a completely irregular and ineffective way (ventricular fibrillation). In neither case is there any circulation of blood. The difference is important only when a doctor or paramedical person is available to apply specialized corrective treatment, and in any case cannot be diagnosed without an electrocardiogram (ECG). The techniques of resuscitation are the same for either form of cardiac arrest.

Cardiac arrest may be due to:

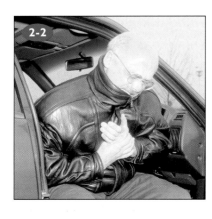

- direct damage to the heart muscle such as occurs during a heart attack (coronary thrombosis) (Figure 2-2) or from an electric shock; or
- failure of the heart muscle to work due to lack of oxygen, such as occurs with prolonged suffocation from any of the causes mentioned above.

If a casualty stops breathing or suffers a cardiac arrest, it is only a short time before he dies from lack of oxygen. The brain is the most sensitive part of the body; within seconds of the heart stopping consciousness will

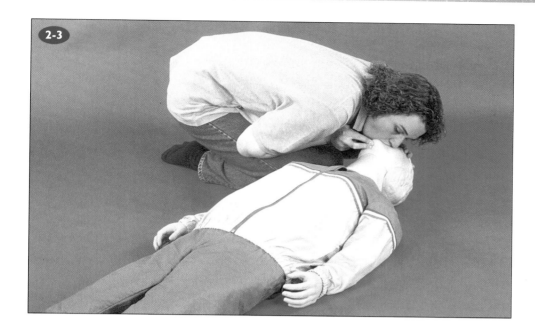

2-3

be lost and within a few minutes death will occur. Life support must be started as soon as possible.

The two main techniques involved in life support are rescue breathing and chest compression.

Rescue Breathing

Rescue Breathing is a technique for providing a non-breathing casualty with the oxygen he or she needs. It is sometimes also called 'the kiss of life' or 'expired air ventilation' and has been shown to be much more effective than any other technique of artificial ventilation that does not rely on special equipment. Basically, it consists of the rescuer blowing air into the casualty's lungs by applying her mouth to the casualty's mouth or nose (Figure 2-3). Although the air which the rescuer blows into the casualty's lungs contains only 17% oxygen compared with 21% in the atmosphere, this is still enough to keep the casualty alive. Even if the casualty is still breathing weakly, rescue breathing is harmless and may well be beneficial.

Rescue breathing can be taught easily to all age groups but its one main drawback is that it can be unpleasant for the rescuer. It is usual to teach the mouth to mouth technique as the preferred option, but some people find the mouth to nose technique more acceptable; the two methods have been shown to be equally effective.

Chest Compression

Chest Compression will maintain circulation of the blood when the heart has stopped and can sometimes stimulate it into beating again (Figure 2-4). The technique consists of rhythmical compressions of the casualty's chest, achieved by the rescuer pressing down on the sternum (breastbone). There is some risk of damage to the heart, chest wall, and abdominal organs during chest compression but this risk is far outweighed by its lifesaving potential.

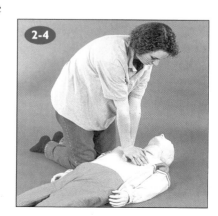

2-4

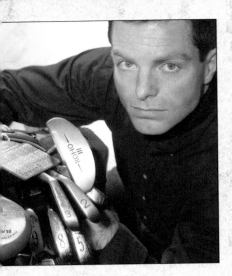

Even the most effective cardiopulmonary resuscitation is only a means of buying time before qualified medical aid arrives. Getting help is always the first priority.

"I owe my life to Ashley," admits Peter Bowyer. "I was enjoying a golf lesson when I collapsed. The last thing I remember was a wave of dizziness and a crushing pain across my chest.

If Ashley hadn't gone for help first, then put his life support training into practice, I'd never have made it."

It is important to remember that chest compression and rescue breathing, even when applied skilfully, may not result in the casualty's recovery. Chest compression and rescue breathing are often only a means of 'buying time' until other medical procedures, particularly electrical defibrillation and more advanced life support techniques, can be applied (Figure 2-5). It is therefore vital to summon help as soon as possible. Each of the elements needed for successful resuscitation can be thought of as links in a 'Chain of Survival' (Figure 2-6).

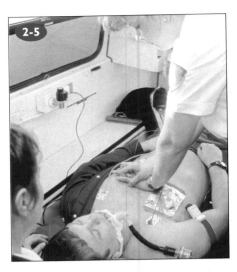

Early access means calling the emergency services (particularly an ambulance) as soon as possible in order to get professional help on its way.

Early basic life support requires those who are present when a casualty has a cardiac arrest (heart stops beating) or stops breathing, to be able and willing to start life support.

Early defibrillation is a technique of applying a controlled electric shock across the chest to re-start the heart. Defibrillators are carried by most emergency ambulances in the UK and, increasingly, are being provided in areas where there is an increased risk of someone having a heart attack.

Early advanced life support includes various medical and paramedical procedures, including injecting drugs into a vein and using specialized artificial ventilation equipment.

It must be appreciated, however, that if too much damage has occurred to the heart or if there has been an unavoidable delay before resuscitation has been started, the casualty may not recover. But if rescuers have applied the techniques of life support correctly and carefully, they should have no cause for self-criticism whatever the outcome.

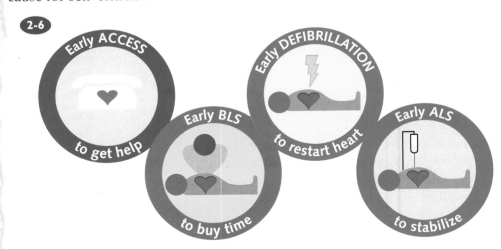

Early ACCESS to get help
Early BLS to buy time
Early DEFIBRILLATION to restart heart
Early ALS to stabilize

Adult Basic Life Support

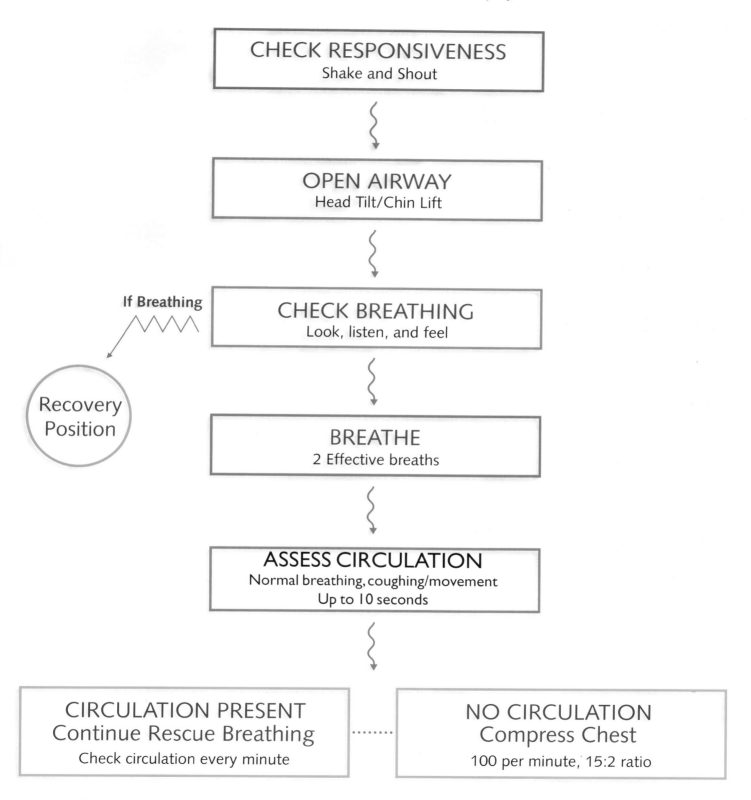

CHECK RESPONSIVENESS
Shake and Shout

OPEN AIRWAY
Head Tilt/Chin Lift

If Breathing

CHECK BREATHING
Look, listen, and feel

Recovery
Position

BREATHE
2 Effective breaths

ASSESS CIRCULATION
Normal breathing, coughing/movement
Up to 10 seconds

CIRCULATION PRESENT
Continue Rescue Breathing
Check circulation every minute

NO CIRCULATION
Compress Chest
100 per minute, 15:2 ratio

Send or go for help as soon as possible according to guidelines on page 27.

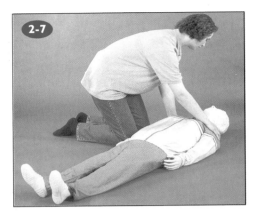

Sequence of Life Support

1 **Ensure safety of rescuer and casualty.**

2 **Check the casualty and see if he responds.**

Gently shake his shoulders and ask loudly:
"Are you all right?" (Figure 2-7)

3A **If the casualty responds by answering or moving:**

Leave him in the position in which you find him (provided
he is not in further danger), check his condition and get help if needed.
   Reasses him regularly.

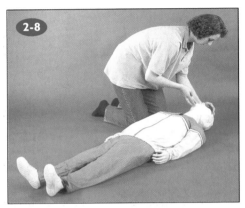

3B **If the casualty does NOT respond:**

Shout for help.
   Unless you can assess him fully in the position you find him,
turn the casualty on to his back and then open the airway.
   Place your hand on his forehead and gently tilt his head back
keeping your thumb and index finger free to close his nose if rescue
breathing is required (Figure 2-8)
   Remove any visible obstruction from the casualty's mouth,
including dislodged dentures, but leave well fitting dentures in place.
   With your fingertip(s) under the point of the casualty's chin,
lift the chin to open the airway.
   **Try to avoid head tilt if trauma (injury) to the neck is
suspected or the casualty is a baby.**

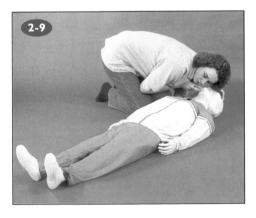

4 Keeping the casualty's airway open, look, listen, and feel for normal
breathing (more than an occasional gasp or weak attempts
at breathing) (Figure 2-9).

Look for chest movement.

Listen at the casualty's mouth for breath sounds.

Feel for air on your cheek.

   Look, listen, and feel for **10 seconds** before deciding
that breathing is absent.

5A **If the casualty IS breathing normally:**

Turn him into the recovery position (page 28)
(Figure 2-10). (See also page 46.)
   Check for continued breathing.

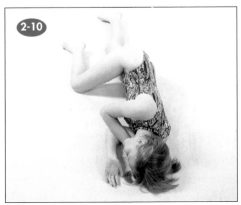

5B If the casualty is **NOT** breathing, or is only making occasional gasps or weak attempts at breathing:

Send someone for help. If you are on your own, leave the casualty and go for help; return and start rescue breathing (see also 'To call for help' page 27).

- Turn the casualty onto his back if he is not already in this position.

- Ensure head tilt and chin lift.

- Give **two slow, effective** rescue breaths, each of which should make the chest rise and fall.

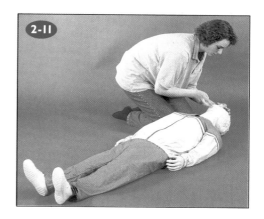

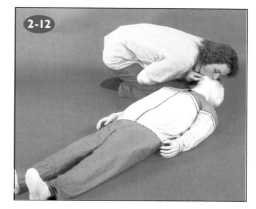

With an adult pinch the soft part of his nose closed with the index finger and thumb of your hand on his forehead (Figure 2-11).

Open his mouth a little but maintain chin lift.

Take a deep breath to fill your lungs with oxygen and place your lips around his mouth, making sure that you have a good seal (Figure 2-12).

For a baby, place your lips over his mouth <u>and</u> nose (Figure 2-14).

Blow steadily into the casualty's mouth whilst watching his chest; take about 2 seconds to make his chest rise as in normal breathing.

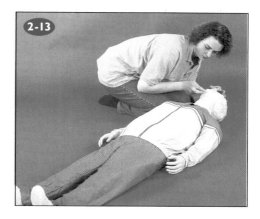

Maintaining head tilt and chin lift, take your mouth away from the casualty and watch for his chest to fall as air comes out (Figures 2-13 and 2-15).

Take another breath and repeat the sequence as above to give two effective rescue breaths in all.

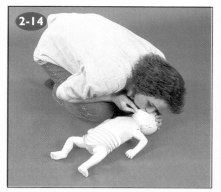

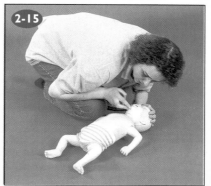

A '**baby**' is defined, for the purposes of resuscitation, as in the first year of life (nappy stage).

A '**child**' is considered to be up to the age of about 8 years.

Turning a Casualty onto the Back

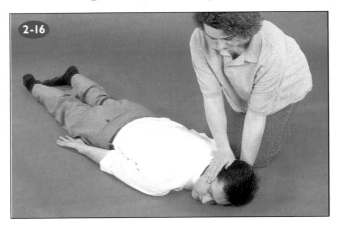

1. Kneel by the casualty's side and turn his head to face away from you; (Figure 2-16)

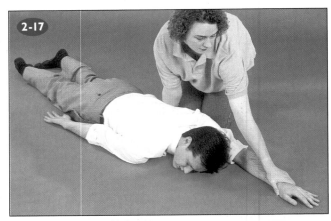

2. Place the arm nearest to you above his head; (Figure 2-17)

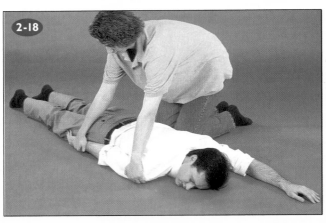

3. With one hand grasp the casualty's far shoulder and with your other hand clamp his wrist to his hip; (Figure 2-18)

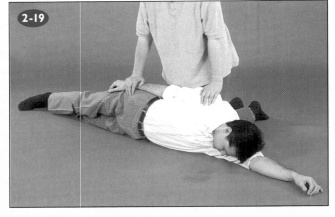

4. With a steady pull roll the casualty over against your thighs; (Figure 2-19)

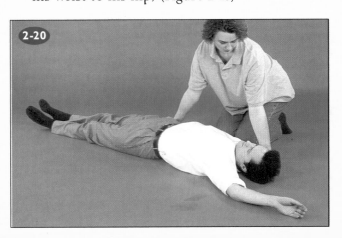

5. Lower the casualty gently to the ground on his back, supporting his head and shoulders as you do so; (Figure 2-20)

Place the casualty's extended arm by his side.

It is important to turn the casualty over as quickly as possible, taking great care not to injure his head.

Only a small amount of resistance to breathing should be felt during rescue breathing and each breath should take about 2 seconds. If you try and blow in too quickly, resistance will be greater and less air will get into the lungs.

You should aim to blow into the casualty's lungs until the chest rises as in normal breathing. **Do not** try to empty your own lungs completely.

Wait for the casualty's chest to fall fully as the air comes out before giving another breath – this should normally take about 2 to 4 seconds, but rather less in a **baby or child**. The exact timing of the air coming out is not critical; wait for the chest to fall, then give another breath.

If you have difficulty achieving an effective breath:

- Recheck the casualty's mouth and remove any obstruction.

- Recheck that there is adequate head tilt and chin lift; **avoid excessive head tilt in babies.**

- **Make up to 5 attempts in all to achieve 2 effective breaths.**

- Even if unsuccessful, move on to assessment of the circulation as described in step 6 below.

If the casualty is a baby or child and you are unable to achieve ANY effective breaths, assume that the airway is obstructed and carry out the actions for choking (See Chapter 3).

6 Assess the casualty for signs of a circulation.

Look, listen and feel for normal breathing, coughing, or movement by the casualty (Figure 2-21).
Take no more than 10 seconds to do this.

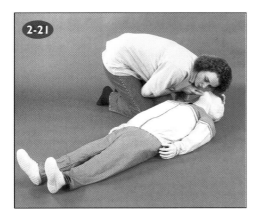

2-21

7A **If you are CONFIDENT that you have detected signs of a circulation:**

Continue rescue breathing until the casualty starts breathing on his own.

About every 10 breaths (or about every minute), check for signs of a circulation; take no more than 10 seconds each time.

If the casualty starts to breathe normally on his own but remains unconscious, turn him into the recovery position. Be ready to turn him onto his back and re-start rescue breathing if he stops breathing.

7B **If there are NO signs of a circulation, or if you are at all unsure:**

Start chest compression, following the procedure below.

To Locate the Correct Position on the Sternum (breastbone)

With your hand that is nearest to the casualty's feet, locate the lower half of the sternum (breastbone):
Using your index and middle fingers, identify the lower rib edge nearest to you. Keeping your fingers together, slide them upwards to the point where the ribs join the sternum. With your middle finger on this point, place your index finger on the sternum itself. (Figure 2-22).

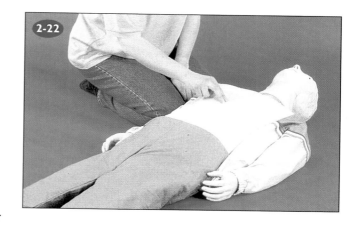

Slide the heel of your other hand down the sternum until it reaches your index finger; this should be the middle of the lower half of the sternum (Figure 2-23).

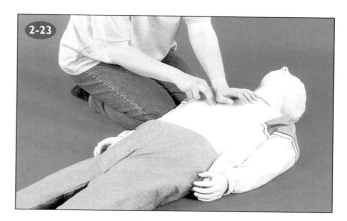

Place the heel of your first hand on top of the one on the sternum.
Extend or interlock the fingers of both hands and lift them to ensure that pressure is not applied over the casualty's ribs. Do not apply any pressure over the upper abdomen or bottom tip of the sternum (Figure 2-24).

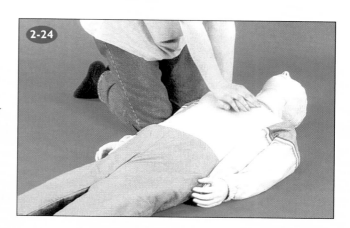

For a baby, imagine a line joining the nipples and place two fingers just below the mid-point of this line (Figure 2-25).

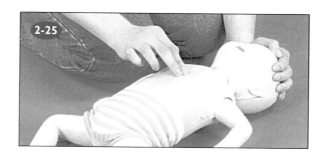

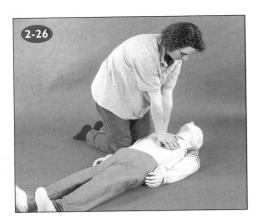

Position yourself vertically above the casualty's chest and, with your arms straight, press down on the sternum to depress it by between 4 and 5 cm (Figure 2-26).

Release the pressure without losing contact between the hand and sternum, then repeat at a rate of about 100 times a minute (a little less than 2 compressions a second); it may be helpful to count out aloud, "1 and-2 and-3 and... 12 and-13-14-15". Compression and release should take an equal amount of time.

At all times the pressure should be firm, controlled and applied vertically; erratic or violent action is dangerous.

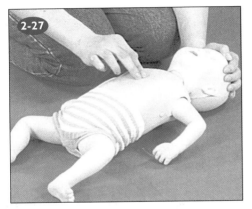

For a baby, use two fingertips only and for a child use one hand (provided sufficient compression can be achieved), compressing to about one-third the depth of the chest (Figure 2-27).

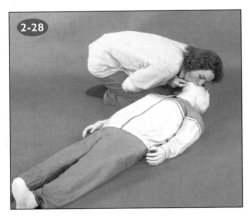

Combine rescue breathing and compression.

After 15 compressions tilt the head, lift the chin and give two effective breaths (Figure 2-28).

Return your hands without delay to the correct position on the sternum and give 15 further compressions, continuing compressions and breaths in a ratio of 15:2.

For a baby or child use a ratio of 5 compressions to 1 rescue breath.

Note: It is essential to combine chest compression with rescue breathing in order that the blood which is being artificially circulated contains adequate amounts of oxygen.

8 Continue Life Support until:

- qualified help arrives (Figure 2-29); or
- the casualty shows signs of life; or
- you become so exhausted that you risk becoming a casualty yourself.

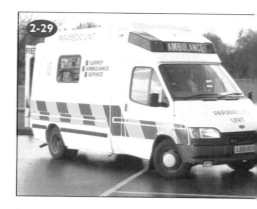

As the chances are remote that effective spontaneous heart action will be restored by chest compression without other techniques of advanced life support (particularly defibrillation), only stop to recheck for signs of a circulation if the casualty makes a movement or takes a spontaneous breath; otherwise life support should not be interrupted.

To Call for Help

It is vital to call for help as quickly as possible. The most effective way of calling for help is to dial 999 (or 112) on any telephone. When the emergency operator answers, ask for the ambulance service. Be ready to give your name, the number you're calling from, the exact location of the emergency and details of the casualty's condition.

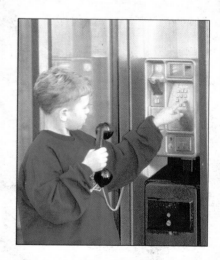

If more than one rescuer is available, one should start life support while another rescuer calls the emergency services.

A lone rescuer will have to decide whether to start life support or go for help first. In these circumstances, if the likely cause of unconsciousness is:

- trauma (injury);

- drowning,

- drug or alcohol intoxication;

- choking; or

- if the casualty is a baby or child,

the rescuer should give life support for about **one minute** before going for help. If the casualty is an **adult** and the cause of unconsciousness is **not** injury, drowning or intoxication, the rescuer should assume that the casualty has a heart problem and go for help as soon as it is established that he is not breathing.

Recovery Position

An unconscious casualty whose airway is clear, and who is breathing spontaneously, should be turned into the recovery position. This prevents the tongue falling back to block the airway, and reduces the risk of stomach contents coming up into the throat and going down into the lungs.

- Remove the casualty's spectacles (if worn)

- Kneel beside the casualty and make sure that both her legs are straight (Figure 2-30).

- Place the arm nearest to you out at right angles to her body, elbow bent, with the hand palm uppermost.

- Bring the far arm across the chest, and hold the back of the hand against the casualty's nearest cheek (Figure 2-31).

- With your other hand, grasp the far leg just above the knee and pull it up, keeping the foot on the ground (Figure 2-32).

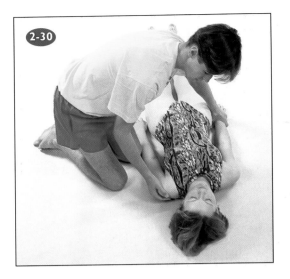

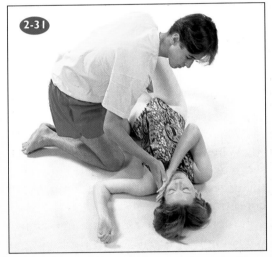

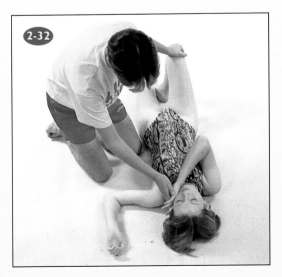

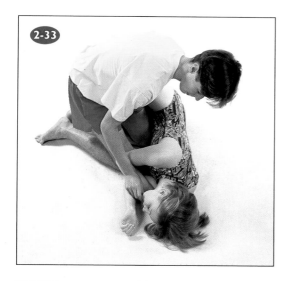

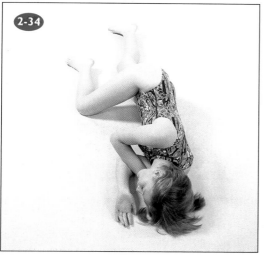

- Keeping her hand pressed against her cheek, pull on the leg to roll the casualty towards you onto her side (Figure 2-33).

- Adjust the upper leg so that both the hip and knee are bent at right angles.

- Tilt the head back to make sure the airway remains open.

- Adjust the hand under the cheek, if necessary, to keep the head tilted (Figure 2-34).

- Check breathing.

Care should be taken to monitor the peripheral circulation of the lower arm, and to ensure that the duration for which there is pressure on this arm is kept to a minimum. If the casualty has to be kept in the recovery position for **more than 30 minutes** she should be turned to the opposite side.

Two Person Life Support

When two or more rescuers are present at a resuscitation attempt they can take turns to perform single person life support. If at least two are trained and proficient in two person life support, for instance when lifeguards are attending a casualty, such a technique has definite advantages in that it results in less interruption to chest compression (Figure 2-35 and 2-36).

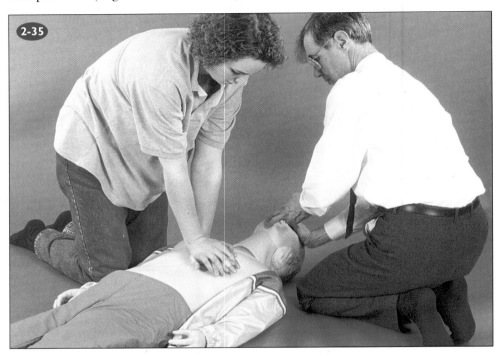

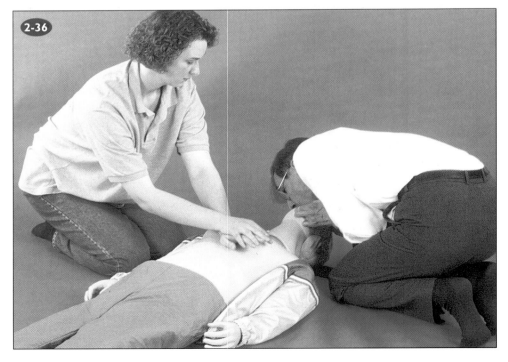

Initially, single person life support may be undertaken while one of the rescuers goes for help, but on his return this can be changed to two person, which is the preferred method, provided both rescuers are trained and proficient in the technique. One rescuer should undertake chest compression while the other gives the rescue breaths. A ratio of 15 compressions to 2 breaths should be used.

When using two person life support the following points should be noted:

- The first priority is to summon help. This may mean that one rescuer has to start resuscitation alone whilst the other leaves to find a telephone.

- When changing from single person to two person life support, the second rescuer should take over chest compression after the first rescuer has given 2 breaths. During these breaths, the incoming rescuer should determine the correct position on the sternum and should be ready to start compressions immediately after the second breath has been given. It is preferable that the rescuers work from opposite sides of the casualty (Figure 2-37).

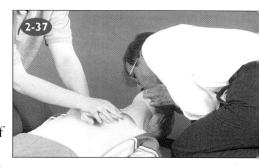

- A ratio of 15 compressions to 2 breaths should be used. By the end of each series of 15 compressions, the rescuer responsible for rescue breathing should be positioned ready to give 2 breaths with the least possible delay. It is helpful if the rescuer giving compressions counts out aloud: "...1 and-2 and-3 and... 12 and-13-14-15".

- Head tilt and chin lift should be maintained at all times. Each rescue breath should take the usual 2 seconds during which chest compressions should cease; they should be resumed immediately after the second breath, waiting only for the rescuer to remove his lips from the casualty's face.

- If the rescuers wish to change places, usually because the one giving compressions becomes tired, this should be undertaken as quickly and smoothly as possible. The rescuer responsible for compressions should announce the change and, at the end of a series of 15 compressions, move rapidly to the casualty's head, obtain an open airway, and give 2 breaths. During this manoeuvre the second rescuer should position himself to commence compressions as soon as the rescue breaths have been completed.

Two person life support may be carried out on babies or children, assuming that both rescuers are trained in the technique. It can, however, sometimes be physically difficult due to the small size of the casualty.

Babies and Children

When carrying out resuscitation of babies or children, the techniques of rescue breathing and chest compression are similar to those for an adult, modified to allow for the difference in size and maturity of the casualty. These differences are highlighted in the appropriate sections in the 'Sequence of Life Support' (page 21).

It is rare for a baby's or a child's heart to stop unexpectedly (cardiac arrest). Problems with the airway and breathing, however, are far more common and, if not treated rapidly and correctly, may lead to cardiac arrest due to lack of oxygen in the blood. Because heart attacks, a major cause of cardiac arrest in adults, are so rare in babies and children, particular attention must be given to obtaining a clear airway in any baby or child whose heart has stopped or who has stopped breathing. This may include action to relieve choking.

In babies and children, breathing may become obstructed or stop because of:

- inhalation of vomit, regurgitated food; or a foreign body such as a small toy or peanut;
- submersion in water (near drowning);
- infection of the throat (croup) or lungs (pneumonia);
- injuries to the head, neck, or chest; or
- sudden infant death syndrome (cot death).

Variation in Resuscitation Techniques

Because of the greater likelihood of a breathing problem in baby or child than in an adult, the rescuer who is on his or her own should undertake about **one minute** of resuscitation (rescue breathing or combined rescue breathing and chest compression as appropriate) before leaving the casualty to go for help (see 'to Call for Help' page 27).

As with adults, rescue breathing should aim to cause the chest to rise and fall as in normal breathing. For babies, the rescuer's mouth should be placed over the casualty's mouth and nose; for a child, normal mouth to mouth rescue breathing is appropriate.

In babies and children it may be difficult to maintain the casualty in a normal recovery position. The aim should be to keep the casualty on his side, maintaining an open airway and allowing vomit to drain freely from the mouth.

A **'baby'** is defined, for the purposes of resuscitation, as in the first year of life (nappy stage).

A **'child'** is considered to be up to the age of about 8 years.

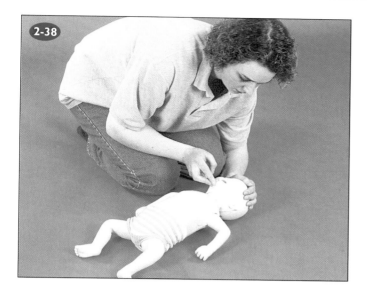

Chest Compression on a Baby

- Put the casualty on a firm surface on his back (Figure 2-38).

- Locate the correct position on the chest by imagining a line joining the nipples and placing two fingers on the sternum (breastbone) just below the mid point of this line.

- Use two fingertips only, compressing to about one third the depth of the chest (Figure 2-39).

- Give compressions and rescue breaths in a ratio of 5 compressions to 1 breath.

It may be possible to obtain sufficient support with your arm behind the baby's back to undertake efficient chest compression (Figure 2-40) while going yourself to the telephone to summon help.

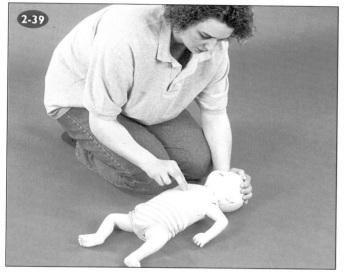

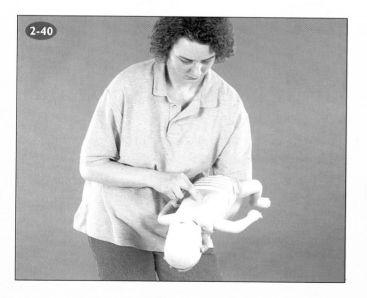

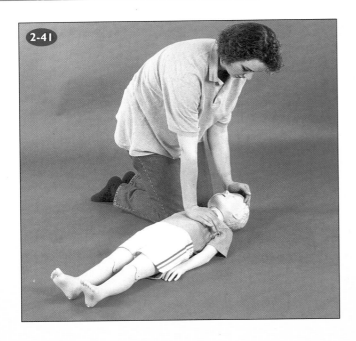

2-41

Chest Compression on Children

- Put the casualty on a firm surface on his back.
- Find the correct position on the chest as you would for an adult.
- Use only one hand, compressing to about one third the depth of the chest (Figure 2-41).
- Give compressions and rescue breaths in a ratio of five compressions to one breath.

Chest compression on a older child (over the age of about 8 years).

- Find the correct position on the chest as you would for an adult.
- Use a depth of compression according to the size of the child, up to the adult figure of 4-5cms (1 to 2 inches).
- As the adult depth of compression is reached, two hands will be needed on the chest and at this point change from a ratio of five compressions to one breath, to a ratio of 15 compressions to 2 breaths.

Difficulties During Life Support Actions

Tracheostomy

Very rarely, a lifesaver may be faced with having to resuscitate a person who has undergone an operation for the removal of the voice box (laryngectomy). This will leave an opening to the windpipe (stoma) in the front of the neck. To carry out rescue breathing:

- Remove stoma cover - do not remove any tube that is in place;
- Wipe any mucus from the stoma or tube;
- Close the casualty's nose and mouth;
- Place your mouth around the opening in his neck; and
- Blow in through the stoma, watching the chest rise and fall as in the mouth to mouth technique.

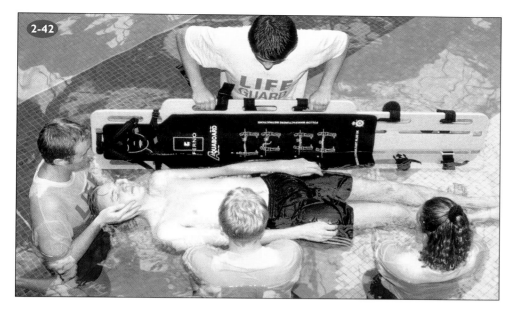

Injury to Spine

If injury to the spine is suspected, for example if the casualty has sustained a fall, been struck on the head or neck, or has been rescued after diving into shallow water, particular care must be taken during handling and resuscitation to maintain alignment of the head, neck and chest. Additional rescuers are often needed.

A spinal board or cervical (neck) collar may be used if either is available, and if the rescuers are trained in its use (Figure 2-42).

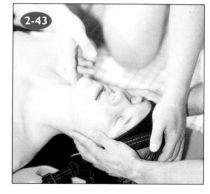

As a fall in blood pressure often accompanies spinal cord injury, care should be taken to maintain the casualty in a horizontal position during rescue.

When opening the airway, head tilt may be used, but the tilt should be the minimum that allows unobstructed rescue breathing (Figure 2-43).

Remember – successful resuscitation which results in paralysis is a tragedy, but failure to get oxygen into the casualty who is not breathing will result in death.

Vomiting

This commonly occurs during or immediately following successful resuscitation. The danger is that stomach contents will enter the air passages and lungs, not only interfering with breathing, but subsequently causing a particularly severe form of pneumonia. Immediate action is essential:

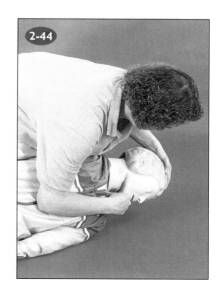

- Turn the casualty away from you. Keep him on his side and use your elbow and forearm to prevent him toppling on to his front;
- Ensure that his head is turned towards the floor and his mouth is open and at the lowest point, thus allowing vomit to drain away (Figure 2-44);
- Clear any residual debris from his mouth with your fingers; and
- Immediately turn him on to his back, re-establish an airway, and continue rescue breathing at the normal rate.

Air in Stomach

If head tilt and chin lift are not adequate to produce a clear airway, extra force will be needed during rescue breathing to blow air past the obstruction. This may drive air down the oesophagus (gullet) into the stomach. As the stomach becomes distended it interferes with the downward movement of the diaphragm and further interferes with air entering the lungs. There is also an increased risk that the casualty may vomit.

If distension of the stomach is seen (a swelling appearing in the abdomen below the left lower ribs):

- Attempt to improve the casualty's airway by increasing head tilt and chin lift if possible; but
- Do not apply pressure over the stomach as this is very likely to induce vomiting. Provided a clear airway is maintained the air in the stomach is likely gradually to escape.

Broken Ribs

During chest compression one or more ribs may be heard to break. In elderly people, or those with particularly rigid chests, this may be unavoidable. It is far more likely to occur if the force used to compress the sternum is excessive, or if the hands are incorrectly placed on the sternum with pressure no longer being applied directly downwards towards the spine. If a rib does break, no action should or can be taken during resuscitation, which should continue uninterrupted. After recovery, the casualty may be expected to be in some pain.

Chapter Two — Test Yourself

1. When might you need to perform life support actions?
2. Give two examples of causes of suffocation.
3. What is cardiac arrest?
4. What can cause cardiac arrest?
5. How does rescue breathing work?
6. What is chest compression?
7. Do rescue breathing and chest compression always work?
8. What are the links in the Chain of Survival?
9. Describe the sequence of life support.
10. What do you do if the casualty responds when you talk to him?
11. When should you shout for help?
12. How do you ensure the casualty's airway is open?
13. When should you avoid tilting the casualty's head?
14. How do you check if the casualty is breathing?
15. Describe how you would give the first two rescue breaths to:
    • an adult casualty;
    • a baby.
16. What signs of a circulation should you look for?
17. How do you perform chest compressions on:
    • an adult?
    • a child?
    • a baby?
18. If you are on your own, when should you leave the casualty to go for help?
19. When should you stay and perform life support?
20. How long should you continue to perform resuscitation?
21. Why should you place an unconscious casualty in the recovery position?
22. Who should perform two person life support?
23. Give some reasons why babies and children may stop breathing.
24. How would you perform rescue breathing on a casualty who has had a tracheostomy?
25. How should you treat a casualty with suspected spinal injury?
26. What should you do if a casualty vomits?
27. How would you deal with air in a casualty's stomach?

3

Lifesaving First Aid

Contents

Choking
    Diagnosis   40
    Treatment   40

Bleeding
    Diagnosis   45
    Treatment   45

Unconscious Breathing Casualties
    Diagnosis   46
    Treatment   46

Shock
    Causes of Shock   48
    Diagnosis   48
    Treatment   48

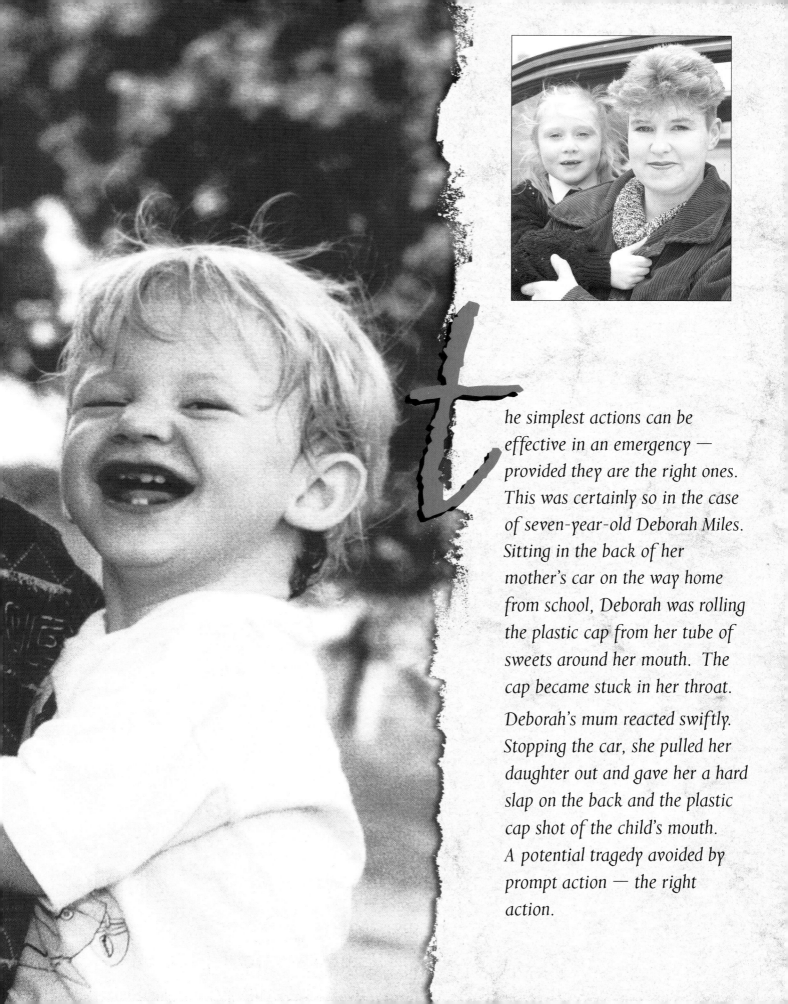

*t*he simplest actions can be effective in an emergency — provided they are the right ones. This was certainly so in the case of seven-year-old Deborah Miles. Sitting in the back of her mother's car on the way home from school, Deborah was rolling the plastic cap from her tube of sweets around her mouth. The cap became stuck in her throat.

Deborah's mum reacted swiftly. Stopping the car, she pulled her daughter out and gave her a hard slap on the back and the plastic cap shot of the child's mouth. A potential tragedy avoided by prompt action — the right action.

Lifesaving and First Aid

{ *uffocation and cardiac arrest are not*

the only life threatening conditions.

Lifesavers need additional skills.

Choking

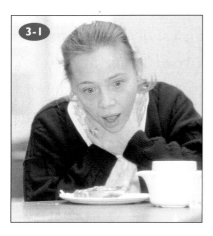

3-1

Choking occurs when a piece of food or other material is swallowed but goes down the trachea (windpipe) rather than the oesophagus (gullet). This results in blockage of the airway. If this blockage is only partial, the casualty will usually be able to dislodge it by coughing. But if there is complete obstruction of the flow of air, coughing may not be possible. Unless help is given urgently the casualty will suffer from suffocation, become unconscious and may die. Even a small piece of food such as a peanut may cause serious obstruction because its presence can lead to muscle spasm in the region of the larynx (voice box). (Figure 3-1)

Diagnosis

- The casualty may have been seen to be eating.
- A child may have been seen putting an object into its mouth.
- A casualty who is choking often grips the throat with one or both hands.
- With **partial airway obstruction** the casualty will be distressed and coughing. Breathing may be noisy (wheezy).
- If the airway is **completely obstructed,** the casualty will be unable to speak, breathe or cough. His face may become blue and congested with the veins standing out in the neck.

Treatment

If the casualty is breathing, encourage coughing but do nothing else.

If the casualty shows signs of becoming weak or stops breathing or coughing, remove any obvious debris or loose false teeth from the mouth and carry out **back slapping** as described on opposite page. This should be done with the casualty in the position in which you found him. The aim is to relieve the obstruction with each slap rather than necessarily to give all five.

- Stand to the side and slightly behind him.

- Support his chest with one hand and lean him well forwards so that when the obstruction is dislodged it comes out of the mouth rather than goes further down the airway.

- Give **up to five** sharp slaps between the shoulder blades with the heel of your other hand (Figure 3-2).

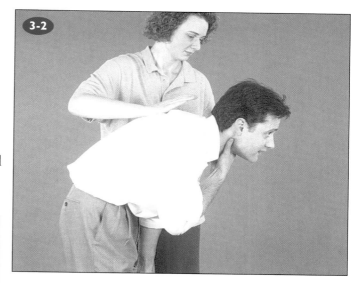

Abdominal Thrusts

If back slapping fails, try giving **abdominal thrusts.** This forces air out of the windpipe by a sudden inward and upward movement of the diaphragm.

- Stand behind the casualty and put both arms round the upper part of his abdomen (Figure 3-3).

- Make sure the casualty is bending well forwards so that when the obstruction is dislodged it comes out of the mouth rather than goes further down the airway.

- Clench your fist and place it just below the point where the lower ribs meet; grasp it with your other hand.

- Pull sharply inwards and upwards. The obstruction should be dislodged and fly out of the mouth.

- If the obstruction is still not relieved, repeat the action, giving up to five abdominal thrusts.

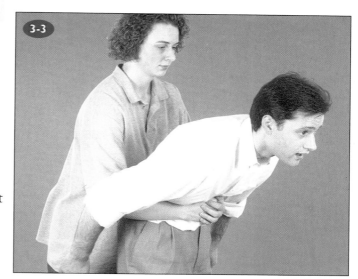

If the casualty at any time becomes unconscious or falls to the ground:

Loss of consciousness may result in relaxation of the muscles around the throat and allow air to pass down into the lungs. If at any time the choking casualty loses consciousness or falls to the ground, follow the **sequence of life support below**. In summary:

- Tilt the casualty's head and remove any visible obstruction from the mouth.

- Open his airway by lifting his chin.

- Check for breathing by looking, listening and feeling.

- Send for help; if you are on your own, do not go at this stage.

- Attempt to give 2 effective rescue breaths:

  - if effective breaths **can** be achieved, continue rescue breathing as appropriate

  - if effective breaths **cannot** be achieved after 5 attempts, start chest compression. **Do not check for signs of a circulation.**

- Give 15 chest compressions then try 5 further attempts at rescue breathing.

- Continue with this sequence.

- If you are on your own, continue for about one minute before leaving the casualty to go for help. Return and resume your efforts.

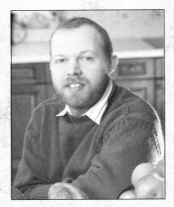

When Alan found himself choking at dinner one evening. He couldn't breathe or speak. Mrs Newhouse kept her head however. Leaning Alan forward, she slapped him hard between the shoulder blades several times but to no avail. She then tried an abdominal thrust.

Alan's life was saved by her first aid and life support training.

How to Treat Choking in a Baby or Child

When treating choking in a baby or child, it may be easier to support the casualty on your knee when giving back slaps. It is important that the head is lower than chest to make sure that the dislodged object comes out of the mouth.

In a baby it is dangerous to give abdominal thrusts. Instead, if five back slaps fail to relieve the obstruction, give five chest thrusts. These are similar to chest compressions and are given to the same place on the sternum (breastbone). The difference is that each thrust is sharper and more vigorous and each aims to relieve the obstruction rether than all five having to be given. It is important that the baby is on his or her back on a firm surface (wich could be your thigh) and that his head is lower than his chest.

If five back slaps followed by five chest thrusts fail to clear the obstruction, look into the mouth and remove any object seen. Then, with the baby on his or her back, open the airway with head tilt and chin lift, and give two effective breaths. If this cannot be achieved after 5 attempts, repeat the sequence of back slaps and chest thrusts.

Steps for Treating Choking Babies

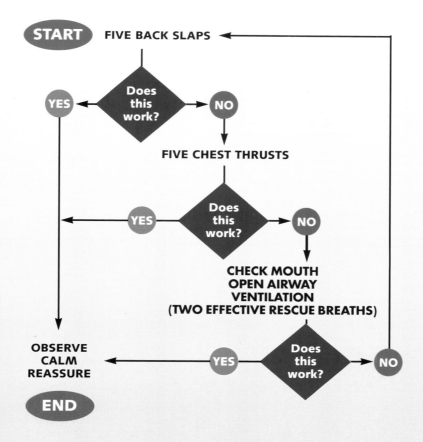

START — FIVE BACK SLAPS

Does this work? — YES — Does this work? — YES — OBSERVE CALM REASSURE — END

NO — FIVE CHEST THRUSTS — Does this work? — NO — CHECK MOUTH OPEN AIRWAY VENTILATION (TWO EFFECTIVE RESCUE BREATHS) — Does this work? — YES — OBSERVE CALM REASSURE

NO

Steps for Treating Choking Children

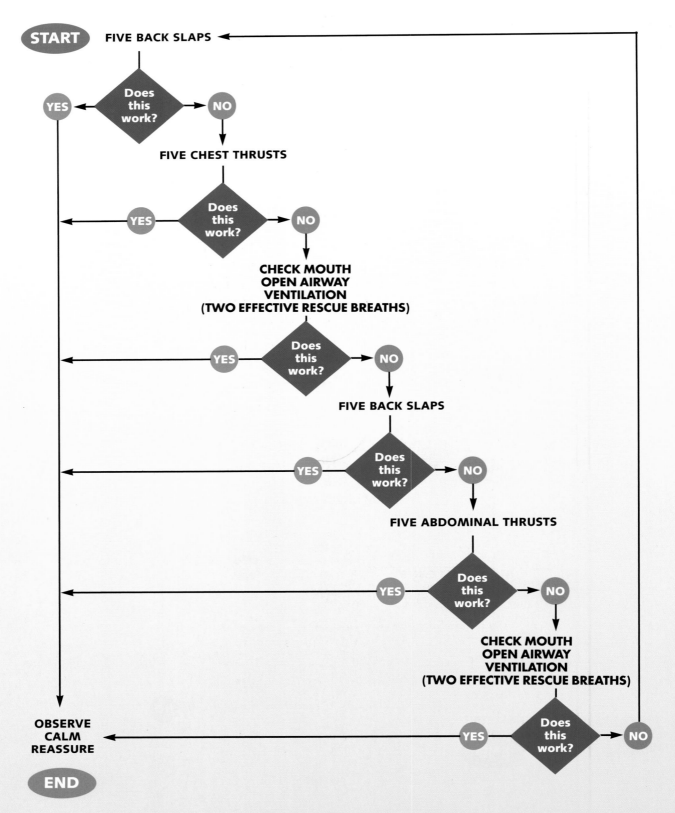

START FIVE BACK SLAPS

Does this work?
YES — NO

FIVE CHEST THRUSTS

Does this work?
YES — NO

CHECK MOUTH
OPEN AIRWAY
VENTILATION
(TWO EFFECTIVE RESCUE BREATHS)

Does this work?
YES — NO

FIVE BACK SLAPS

Does this work?
YES — NO

FIVE ABDOMINAL THRUSTS

Does this work?
YES — NO

CHECK MOUTH
OPEN AIRWAY
VENTILATION
(TWO EFFECTIVE RESCUE BREATHS)

Does this work?
YES — NO

OBSERVE
CALM
REASSURE

END

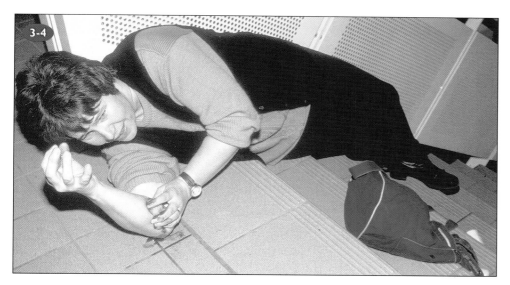

3-4

Bleeding

If blood is lost from the circulation, the amount of oxygen that can be carried to the organs and tissues of the body is reduced. If bleeding is severe it can lead to shock and ultimately to death. Bleeding may occur externally (for example, a cut or graze) (Figure 3-4) or internally (for example, rupture of the spleen after a blow to the abdomen or bleeding into a muscle after a crush injury).

Diagnosis

- **External bleeding** is usually obvious but a quick examination of the whole casualty, including any necessary removal of clothing, will ensure that no hidden bleeding is missed.
- **Internal bleeding** is difficult to diagnose; signs of shock may occur and the casualty should be treated for this condition (see above).

Treatment

Put on protective gloves if these are available.

Apply direct pressure to the wound, preferably using a dressing or pad of clean material; if this is not available use your fingers or the palm of your hand. If the bleeding does not stop, do not remove the dressings, but apply more on top of the first and bandage firmly.

If the wound is long it may be more effective to press the edges together with your fingers. Do this gently but firmly.

If there is an obvious foreign body in the wound do not apply dressings over the foreign body but apply pressure to the edges of the wound.

Lay the casualty down in a comfortable position and raise the injured part if possible. Support it by hand or in a suitable sling.

Treat for shock (See page 47.).

Summon medical assistance or take the casualty to a doctor or hospital. Even if the wound appears minor, further treatment may be necessary to prevent infection.

Bleeding

DIRECT PRESSURE ON WOUND

ELEVATE LIMB

Unconscious Breathing Casualty

CHECK RESPONSIVENESS

OPEN AIRWAY
and CHECK BREATHING

PLACE IN RECOVERY POSITION

OBSERVE

Unconscious Breathing Casualties

Loss of consciousness may be due to:

- a reduced supply of blood to the brain: strangulation, heart attack, shock or fainting;
- temporary or permanent brain injury: head injury, stroke, poisoning or hypothermia;
- disturbance of the normal electrical activity of the brain (epilepsy);
- a reduced amount of oxygen in the blood (suffocation or drowning); or
- an abnormal level of sugar in the blood (diabetes).

Diagnosis

Reduced consciousness may vary from slight drowsiness or confusion to deep coma in which the casualty is totally unresponsive.

For the purpose of deciding on first aid treatment a simple distinction between conscious and unconscious can be made by gently shaking the casualty and calling: "Can you hear me? Open your eyes".

When you do this, be careful not to move the casualty unnecessarily as you could aggravate any injuries, particularly to the neck.

Treatment

Treat any cause of unconsciousness that you can.

Ensure that the casualty's airway is clear using head tilt and chin lift (Figure 3-5).

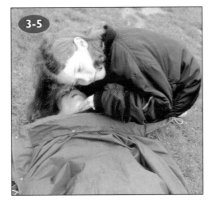

- Place him in the recovery position, taking particular care to move the head and neck as little as possible if you suspect there is a spinal injury.
- Examine the casualty and treat any serious injuries.
- Keep the casualty protected from cold and wet.
- Call or go for further medical help or an ambulance but do not leave the casualty unattended unless you are on your own and have to go for help yourself.
- Maintain observation of the casualty's breathing.
- **Do not** give the casualty anything to eat or drink in case an anaesthetic is needed later because food or drink in the stomach may cause vomiting. Also, an unconscious casualty is unable to swallow food or drink.

Shock

Shock can be defined as 'failure of the circulation which results in an inadequate supply of blood to vital organs.' It occurs when, for a number of reasons, there is not enough blood being pumped round the body. Since one of the main functions of blood is to carry oxygen, failure of the circulation means that essential parts of the body such as the brain, kidneys and heart do not receive as much oxygen as they need and can no longer function properly (Figure 3-6). Unless the casualty is treated quickly and adequately death may result.

Causes of Shock

- Loss of blood volume: external or internal bleeding; loss of fluid from burns; vomiting; diarrhoea; profuse sweating.
- Heart failure (failure of the 'pump'): heart attack; some virus infections; severe irregularity of the heart beat.
- Other causes: blood infections; severe pain; injury; near-drowning.

The body tries to compensate for the lack of circulating blood in three ways:

- by drawing the remaining blood away from the skin and directing it in preference to more important areas;
- by increasing the rate of breathing to get as much oxygen as possible into the blood; and
- by speeding up the heart to circulate the blood more rapidly.

Shock

```
┌─────────────────────────────────────┐
│   CHECK AND TREAT CAUSE              │
└─────────────────────────────────────┘
                 ↓
┌─────────────────────────────────────┐
│   LAY FLAT, ELEVATE LEGS            │
└─────────────────────────────────────┘
                 ↓
┌─────────────────────────────────────┐
│   SEEK HELP URGENTLY                │
└─────────────────────────────────────┘
```

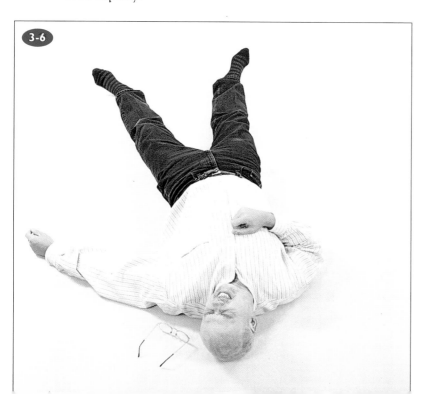

3-6

Diagnosis

The signs of shock are produced by lack of oxygen together with the body's compensating mechanisms.

The brain suffers most from a reduced blood supply, so that a shocked casualty feels faint, dizzy and confused, and in severe cases may become unconscious.

As blood is drawn away from the surface, the skin becomes pale and cold to the touch. Sweating often accompanies shock, but does not appear to have any useful purpose, simply being a reflex response to the reduced blood flow.

The heart speeds up as the reduced volume of blood in the arteries gives rise to a low blood pressure.

Breathing is rapid and the casualty seems to be gasping for air.

Treatment

Treat the cause if possible. Stop any external bleeding; dress burns; reassure the casualty.

- Lay the casualty flat with her legs raised (Figure 3-7), unless she is unconscious, when she should be placed in the recovery position.

- Keep her warm enough to prevent heat loss.

- **Do not** give the casualty anything to eat or drink in case an anaesthetic is needed later because food or drink in the stomach may cause vomiting.

- Get the casualty to hospital as a matter of urgency.

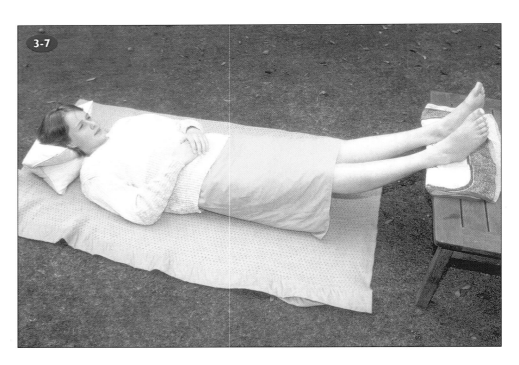

3-7

Chapter Three — Test Yourself

1. How do you recognize that a person is choking?

2. What should you do if the airway is only partially blocked?

3. How do you give back slaps?

4. How do you give abdominal thrusts?

5. List the sequence of actions for a choking adult and for a choking child.

6. How should you deal with a long cut?

7. What should you do if a wound has an obvious foreign body in it?

8. Give some reasons why a casualty might become unconscious.

9. How should you treat an unconscious casualty?

10. What can cause shock?

11. How do you treat a casualty with shock?

4

Drowning, Hypothermia and Life Support

Contents

Drowning   52

Rescue of the Casualty   53

Life Support in the Water   53

   Standing in Shallow Water   54

   On Reaching Support   54

Hypothermia   54

Rescue of the Casualty   55

   Unconscious or Semi-conscious Casualties   56

   Life Support of Cold Casualties   57

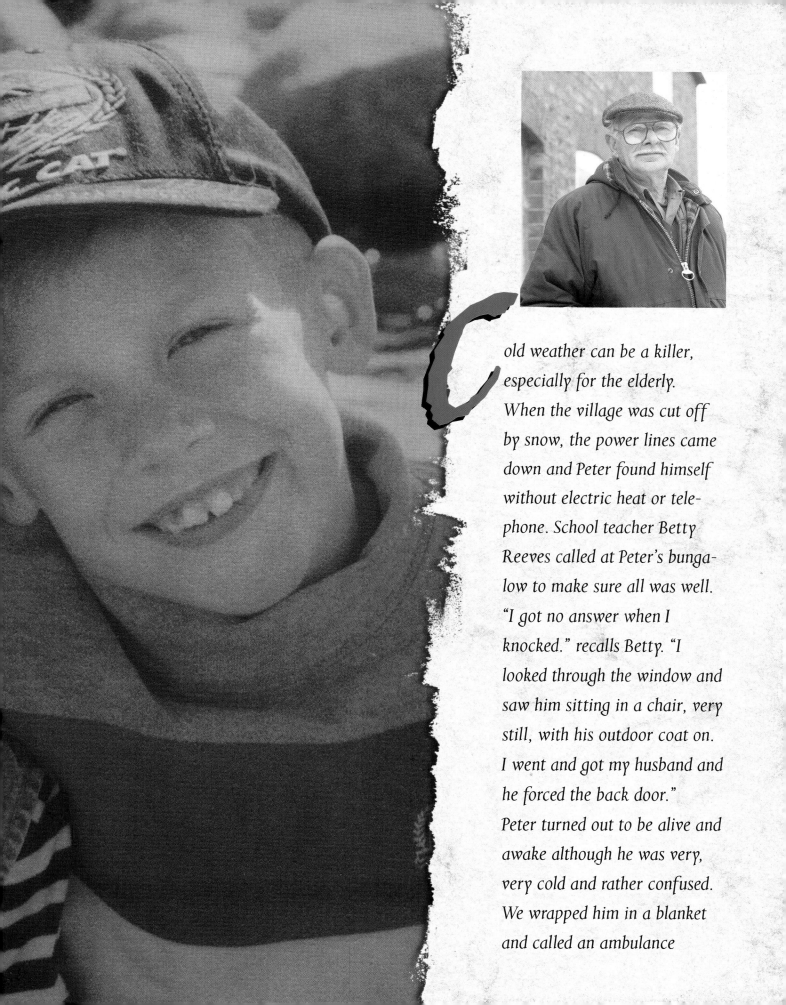

Cold weather can be a killer, especially for the elderly. When the village was cut off by snow, the power lines came down and Peter found himself without electric heat or telephone. School teacher Betty Reeves called at Peter's bungalow to make sure all was well. "I got no answer when I knocked." recalls Betty. "I looked through the window and saw him sitting in a chair, very still, with his outdoor coat on. I went and got my husband and he forced the back door." Peter turned out to be alive and awake although he was very, very cold and rather confused. We wrapped him in a blanket and called an ambulance

Drowning, Hypothermia and Life Support

Drowning is death caused by suffocation following immersion in water. Several hundred people in the British Isles die this way each year. The term 'near-drowning' is used if the casualty survives.

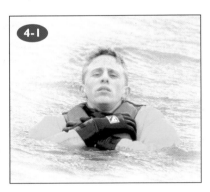

4-1

Drowning

Although the final cause of death is failure of air to get into the lungs, there are often other factors which lead up to this and may therefore be considered causes of drowning (Figure 4-1). For example, a sudden incapacitating illness, such as a stroke or heart attack, may result in someone falling into the water and being unable to get out or swim. The low water temperature around the British coast rapidly produces hypothermia with consequent loss of muscle control and inhalation of water into the lungs. In about one quarter of fatal drowning incidents, alcohol intoxication is a contributory factor.

In most cases of drowning, relatively small quantities of water enter the lungs, but this is enough to interfere with the normal transfer of oxygen to the blood. The water also causes irritation to the lung tissues, and results in an outpouring of fluid from the blood into the lungs which further impairs oxygen transfer. This 'secondary drowning' can be delayed for up to 72 hours, so it is important to watch carefully any immersion victim even if he appears to have recovered fully.

There is little difference between the effect of inhaling small amounts of fresh or sea water. But if a large quantity of water gets into the lungs, fresh water leads to more rapid drowning because it is absorbed into the blood stream and damages the red blood cells.

In about one drowning in ten, water does not get into the lungs because of muscle spasm in the region of the larynx. However, this spasm cuts off the air supply and produces suffocation — so called 'dry drowning'.

If someone is immersed in water for a long time, the pressure of the water on the body has a 'squeezing' effect. Because the volume of the body is made smaller, the normal amount of body fluid (blood and the fluid in and around the body cells) is relatively too great, and some of this is got rid of through the kidneys. When the casualty is rescued, his body re-expands but there is now insufficient blood and fluid to fill the restored volume. As a result, blood circulation becomes inadequate and signs of shock (described in Chapter 3) may appear. This condition is known as 'post-immersion collapse' and was commonly seen after sea rescues during the Second World War.

   An important point to remember is that if someone is rescued from open water (such as the sea, a lake or a reservoir) and is unconscious but has clearly been able to keep his face clear of the water (for example, in a lifejacket), he is more likely to be suffering the effects of cold than near-drowning (see below).

Rescue of the Casualty

The golden rule is to avoid putting your own life at risk — after all, you can't help the casualty if you are in difficulty yourself. Take a few moments to assess the situation. Enlist the assistance of other bystanders if possible. Send someone to summon professional help. Try and effect a rescue by reaching to conscious casualties with a stick, pole, fishing rod, or by throwing them a rope or knotted clothing (Figure 4-2). Only enter the water yourself as a last resort and if you are absolutely sure you will be able to cope (Figure 4-3). Never venture on to ice.

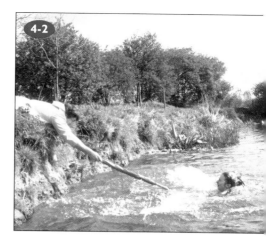

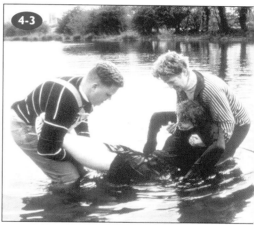

   If possible keep the casualty horizontal during the rescue to counteract shock due to post-immersion collapse and to allow any water and vomit to drain from the mouth.

   Do not attempt to empty water out of the lungs since the little free fluid that is likely to be there is difficult or impossible to get out. There is the added danger that any water expelled will be from the stomach and may then be inhaled into the lungs.

   Turn the casualty on to his back, clear obvious debris from the mouth, and assess the need for rescue breathing or chest compression.

   Drowning casualties often vomit or have froth around their mouths. This makes rescue breathing unpleasant, but the lifesaver **must** be prepared to continue resuscitation under these conditions.

   Do not stop resuscitation even in apparently hopeless cases; complete recovery has been reported after prolonged resuscitation even when the casualty has initially appeared dead.

Life Support in the Water

It is virtually impossible to provide sufficient support behind the casualty's back to carry out chest compression in the water. Rescue breathing is possible while swimming but requires a considerable degree of skill, a powerful swimming stroke and stamina. Rescuers should always try to find some form of support, such as the side of a boat or a floating aid.

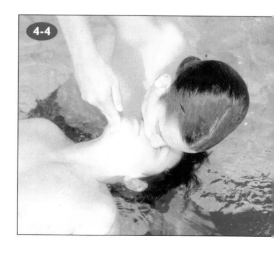

   While giving rescue breathing, the rescuer must try to bring the casualty to shore as quickly as possible in order to carry out more effective resuscitation. The mouth to nose technique is preferable in the water (Figure 4-4) because it frees an arm and hand (used to close the nose in the mouth to mouth technique) to support the casualty and to hold on to the side or a floating rescue aid.

Standing in Shallow Water

- Support the casualty by passing your arm behind his shoulders.
- Quickly remove any debris from the mouth.
- Lift his chin in the usual way. The weight of his legs in the water will assist head tilt.
- Ensure that water does not splash over his face.
- If the casualty is not breathing, give rescue breaths using the mouth to nose technique (see Chapter 2). You can do this while walking through the water to the bank or other point of support.

On Reaching Support

- Support the casualty with one arm passing behind his neck to grip the bank or other means of support.
- Use your other hand to lift the casualty's chin.
- Assess for breathing.
- Unless the casualty starts breathing at once, give two **effective** rescue breaths.
- Then take no more than **10 seconds** to assess the casualty for signs of a circulation (normal breathing, coughing or any movement).
- **If you are confident that you can detect signs of circulation**, continue rescue breathing for a further two or three breaths or until you have recovered from the exertions of towing, then land the casualty, with assistance if available.
- **If there are no signs of a circulation, or you are at all unsure,** land the casualty as quickly as possible (whether help is available or not).
- Once the casualty has been landed, reassess and continue rescue breathing or start chest compression as necessary.
- Ensure that an ambulance has been called.

Hypothermia

Hypothermia (reduced body temperature) is said to exist when the centre (or 'core') of the body falls to a temperature below 35°C. The core temperature does not have to drop as low as this for the casualty to suffer ill effects from the cold, so to avoid confusion with the medical definition of hypothermia the term 'cold casualty' will be used in this chapter.

During exposure to a cold environment, a cold casualty results if the rate of heat being lost from the body exceeds that being produced. This can occur as a result of heat production being overwhelmed by the extreme cold of the environment, for example during immersion in cold water, or from a combination of exhaustion and exposure, which is particularly dangerous; this is classically encountered when people go hill walking in cold weather. Deterioration can then be rapid. People are at particular risk if their clothing is wet or flimsy and a strong wind is blowing.

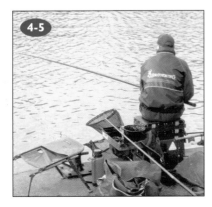
4-5

A cold casualty can also occur in an environment that is only moderately cold (Figure 4-5) if heat production is impaired due to exhaustion or intoxication from drugs or alcohol, or when injury or some accident causes immobilization.

The very old and very young are particularly vulnerable to the cold.

As body cooling may occur only very slowly, an awareness of this potential risk is essential for its prevention, early recognition, and treatment. Early signs may include: shivering; changes in behaviour or personality; slurring of speech; incoordination; stumbling; and slowing of physical and mental activity.

In the situations in which casualties are likely to be suffering the effects of cold (exposure and immersion) it would be unusual for a thermometer, particularly a low reading thermometer, to be available. For practical purposes, therefore, a casualty may be considered to be suffering the effects of cold if his body feels 'as cold as marble' and, in particular, if the armpit is profoundly cold.

Rescue of the Casualty

At all times it is important to ensure the safety of the rescuers as well as the casualty. This becomes particularly important when the casualty is in a hostile environment, such as in the water or on a hillside. Rescuers must ensure that they do not also become casualties from the cold, either through exhaustion or due to loss of insulation as a result of donating their own clothing to the casualty (Figure 4-6).

If the casualty is cold but conscious or only a little confused:

- Lay the casualty flat and undertake any necessary first aid;
- Prevent further heat loss by enclosing the casualty in a sleeping bag if available, or cover with any available material such as a blanket or spare clothing, and include cover for the head. Insulate from the ground and provide overall waterproof and windproof protection if required, for example by using a plastic cover. Once the casualty has been well wrapped, do not disturb him any more than necessary as this risks further heat loss;

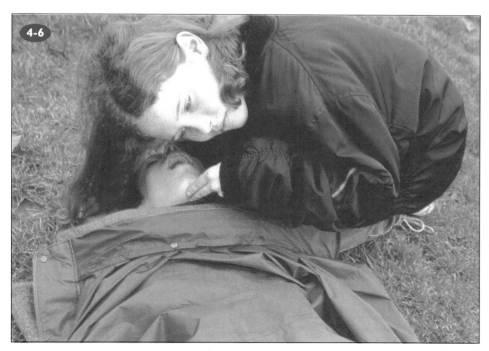

4-6

If evacuation to hospital is not immediately possible and facilities are available, a casualty who is conscious, shivering and uninjured, may be immersed to the neck in a warm bath, provided he can get into it with minimal assistance. The temperature of the bath should be approximately 40°C (which feels comfortable to your own elbow and to the casualty) and should be maintained at this temperature by constantly stirring and adding warm water as necessary. This treatment will require a large supply of warm water.

Heavy outer clothing should be gently removed before the casualty is immersed. Assistance should be given to remove the remaining clothing when the casualty is comfortably settled in the bath.

Shivering will stop almost immediately the casualty is immersed in the warm water but the casualty should stay in the water until he says that he feels comfortably warm. Then help him out of the bath, encourage him to lie flat, and dry and cover him with blankets. Do not allow him to remain in the bath if he complains of feeling hot or starts sweating.

Keep the casualty lying flat until he says he is warm and he feels warm to the touch.

- Provide further protection from the wind and elements by finding or creating shelter if possible. As a temporary measure two rescuers lying either side of a cold casualty and 'hugging' him can be surprisingly effective. If the environment remains cold and hostile, do not attempt to undress the casualty. Instead, insulate and enclose him in a wind and waterproof covering;

- If possible the casualty should be carefully moved, keeping him in a horizontal position (to avoid a drop in blood pressure), to a warmer environment, for example a shelter or house, to reduce further heat loss;

- Once under shelter, if the casualty's clothing is dry he should be kept in blankets or a sleeping bag with cover over his head and allowed to re-warm slowly. If his clothing is wet he should be given assistance to replace his wet clothing with dry;

- Ideally, re-warming should be passive with the heat coming from the core of the body rather than the surface. Even in a warm environment, the casualty should be wrapped in blankets or a sleeping bag to insulate from external heat; there is otherwise a danger that re-warming may occur too quickly from the surface, resulting in a potentially catastrophic fall in blood pressure;

- Consider using a loose scarf to cover the nose and mouth to prevent further loss of heat, provided this does not in any way obstruct the airway;

- Offer a warm sweet drink if available but only if the casualty is able to swallow easily. This will have little effect on raising body temperature but may be comforting. Do not give any alcohol;

- Enquire about co-existing illness such as diabetes, epilepsy, and so on because this information may be valuable to subsequent medical attendants;

- Maintain close observation of the casualty's circulation and respiration; and

- Obtain help as soon as possible and transport the casualty to hospital.

Unconscious or Semi-conscious Casualties

If the casualty is unconscious or semi-conscious and is unable to help himself without assistance, he should be regarded as being in a critical condition. The major aim of treatment should be to prevent further loss of heat and to enable passive re-warming to occur. Try and keep the casualty as still as possible. A hypothermic heart is very 'irritable' and any movement may precipitate cardiac arrest.

Once under shelter the casualty should be carefully wrapped in blankets or a sleeping bag. Wet clothing should only be removed if sufficient rescuers are available to do this with minimum movement of the casualty. This will almost inevitably necessitate cutting some of the clothing.

Carefully place the casualty in the recovery position until he regains consciousness, and then maintain him lying flat until he says that he feels warm, and he feels warm to the touch.

Life Support of Cold Casualties

Normal techniques for rescue breathing and chest compression should be used (see Chapter Two). After the initial two effective breaths of rescue breathing, **up to one minute** may be needed to assess the casualty for signs of a circulation. This length of time is needed because the heart slows down and the body reacts accordingly in profound hypothermia.

The rates for both rescue breathing and chest compression should be the same as for other casualties. It must be recognized, however, that hypothermia may cause stiffness of the chest wall so that more resistance is met. The aims should be to inflate with a volume of air sufficient to cause the chest to rise visibly, and to compress the chest (sternum) to a depth of 4-5 cms in an adult (one third the depth of the chest in a baby or child).

The adverse weather conditions that give rise to a casualty of hypothermia can affect the rescuers as well. Since rescue may take place some considerable distance from help, and there may be no realistic expectation of getting the casualty to a hospital or other medical facility within a reasonable length of time, a decision may need to be made as to whether it is correct to start or continue resuscitation.

Absolute rules cannot be laid down, but as a guide, life support, particularly chest compression, should only be started in a cold casualty if there is a reasonable expectation that it can be provided continuously (or with only brief periods of interruption for movement of the casualty) until that casualty can be transported to a hospital or site where full advanced life support can be provided. In practice, this is likely to mean being within 2 hours travelling time of a suitable hospital.

Remember that life support which cannot be maintained effectively will not help the casualty, and will only serve to exhaust the rescuers and lead in turn to them becoming casualties.

Chapter Four — Test Yourself

1. How is drowning defined?
2. What are 'near-drowning' and 'secondary drowning'?
3. What is post-immersion collapse?
4. How should you counteract shock when rescuing someone from water?
5. Why should you try to resuscitate someone who appears to be dead from drowning?
6. How do you give life support in the water?
7. What is hypothermia?
8. What signs suggest a casualty is feeling the effects of cold?
9. How do you treat a cold casualty?
10. Why should you wrap a cold casualty in blankets in a warm environment?
11. Describe possible problems when giving life support to a cold casualty.

Glossary of Terms

Airway
The passage by which air enters and leaves the lungs

Artery
A tubular vessel which takes blood from the heart to the body or lungs

Asystole
Complete inactivity of the heart

Body core
The central part of the body, away from the surface, including the major organs such as the heart, lungs and liver

Cardiac
Referring to the heart

Cardiac arrest
Cessation of heart beat

Cardiopulmonary resuscitation (CPR)
Combined rescue breathing and chest compression

Cervical
referring to the neck

Chest compression
Rhythmical pressure on the chest to maintain circulation of the blood when the heart has stopped or to relieve an obstruction in a choking adult

Choking
Partial or complete blockage of the upper airway by a particle of food or other foreign body

Contract
Shorten (as of a muscle)

Core temperature
Temperature of the centre of the body or body core

Coronary thrombosis
Blockage of an artery on the surface of the heart by a blood clot, which results in damage to the heart muscle (heart attack)

CPR
Cardiopulmonary resuscitation

Defibrillator
A device for delivering an electric shock to a casualty to correct ventricular fibrillation

Diabetes
A disease in which the body is unable to handle sugar and other carbohydrates correctly

Diaphragm
The dome-shaped muscle which separates the chest from abdomen

Drowning
Death caused by suffocation due to immersion in water

Dry drowning
Drowning in which no water reaches the lungs

Near-drowning
Survival of a casualty after an immersion incident

Secondary drowning
Outpouring of fluid from the blood into the lungs due to irritation by inhaled water

Epilepsy
A condition in which abnormal electrical discharges in the brain produce seizures or fits

Expired air ventilation
Rescue breathing

Fibrillation
See Ventricular fibrillation

First aid
The initial or emergency help given to a casualty before qualified medical assistance arrives

Heart attack
See Coronary thrombosis

Heart failure

Failure of the heart to maintain an adequate circulation of blood

Hypothermia

Reduction of the deep body (core) temperature to below 35°C

Inhale

1) To breathe in
2) To go down the air passages rather than the oesophagus (gullet)

Inspiration

Breathing in

Laryngectomy

Surgical removal of the larynx (voice box), often because of cancer

Larynx

That portion of the airway in the upper neck which contains the vocal cords; the voice box

Oesophagus

A muscular tube which acts as a food passage from the mouth to the stomach; the gullet

Oxygen (O₂)

The gas which is essential for life and makes up about 21% of the air

Pneumonia

Inflammation of the lung, usually caused by an infection

Recovery position

The position in which unconscious casualties are placed to allow observation of their breathing and to prevent obstruction of the airway

Respiration

Breathing
The complete process of getting oxygen to the cells of the body and getting rid of carbon dioxide

Resuscitation

The act of reviving a nearly dead or apparently dead casualty

Shock

Failure of the circulation which results in an inadequate supply of blood to vital organs

Spinal cord

The column of nerve tissue, continuous with the base of the brain, which is protected by the bony spine

Sternum

The flat bone, forming the front of the chest, to which most of the ribs are attached; the breastbone

Suffocation

Obstruction of the airway, preventing an adequate amount of air reaching the lungs

Trachea

The semi-rigid tube, felt in the front of the neck, that takes air from the larynx into the chest; the windpipe

Tracheostomy

A hole made in the trachea (windpipe) to allow breathing when there is obstruction of the upper airway

Vein

A tubular vessel which takes blood from the body or lungs to the heart

Ventricular fibrillation

Irregular, ineffective twitching of the main pumping chambers (ventricles) of the heart which produces no circulation of blood; one form of cardiac arrest

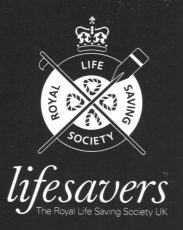

lifesavers
The Royal Life Saving Society UK

The Royal Life Saving Society UK is Britain's leading water safety and drowning prevention organisation. Despite the enormous increase in water based leisure activity, the number of drownings in Britain has steadily declined since our foundation in 1891. However, several hundred people still drown each year. We believe even one drowning is one too many, so the fight to save lives must go on.

Ensuring the safety of swimming pool users is a vital part of our mission and we are the premier provider of training for pool lifeguards. Our National Pool Lifeguard Qualification programme is widely recognised as the professional bench-mark for the sport and leisure industry. We train up to 20,000 swimming pool lifeguards each year and, together with the Surf Life Saving Association of Great Britain, we also train beach lifeguards.

Promoting life support skills in the community is another important aspect of our work. One in three Britons will suffer a heart attack at some time in their life. Our programmes aim to teach resuscitation techniques to those who need them most. We train up to 250,000 members of the public annually and produce a range of training publications.

RLSS UK is a self-financing registered charity. Our work depends upon the dedication of our supporters, members, volunteers and the generosity of benefactors and corporate donors and sponsors.

YOU can help us to save lives. Please use the tear-off form opposite to become a supporter of RLSS UK. Alternatively, write to us for details of full individual membership.

Simply fill in this form

I WISH TO BECOME A SUPPORTER OF RLSS UK
(Annual Fee £6.00)

Title   Mr / Ms / Miss / Mrs / Dr (Delete as appropriate)

Forename(s) _____

Surname _____

Postal Address _____

_____

Post Code _____

AN EASY WAY TO PAY

PLEASE TICK AS APPROPRIATE

I enclose ☐ cheque   ☐ postal order (Payable to RLSS UK)

Please debit my account

I wish to pay by   ☐ Mastercard   ☐ Visa/Delta
                   ☐ Switch

Card No ☐☐☐☐☐☐☐☐☐☐☐☐☐☐☐☐

Issue No ☐☐   Expiri Date ☐☐☐☐   Valid from ☐☐☐☐

Cardholder's Signature

Please send completed form in an envelope addressed to:
FREEPOST (BM 4545), ALCESTER, Warwickshire B50 4BR
(No stamp required if posted in UK or Northern Ireland)

Thank You For Your Support

Simply fill in this form

I WISH TO BECOME A SUPPORTER OF RLSS UK
(Annual Fee £6.00)

Title   Mr / Ms / Miss / Mrs / Dr (Delete as appropriate)

Forename(s) _____

Surname _____

Postal Address _____

_____

Post Code _____

AN EASY WAY TO PAY

PLEASE TICK AS APPROPRIATE

I enclose ☐ cheque   ☐ postal order (Payable to RLSS UK)

Please debit my account

I wish to pay by   ☐ Mastercard   ☐ Visa/Delta
                   ☐ Switch

Card No ☐☐☐☐☐☐☐☐☐☐☐☐☐☐☐☐

Issue No ☐☐   Expiri Date ☐☐☐☐   Valid from ☐☐☐☐

Cardholder's Signature _____

Please send completed form in an envelope addressed to:
FREEPOST (BM 4545), ALCESTER, Warwickshire B50 4BR
(No stamp required if posted in UK or Northern Ireland)

Thank You For Your Support

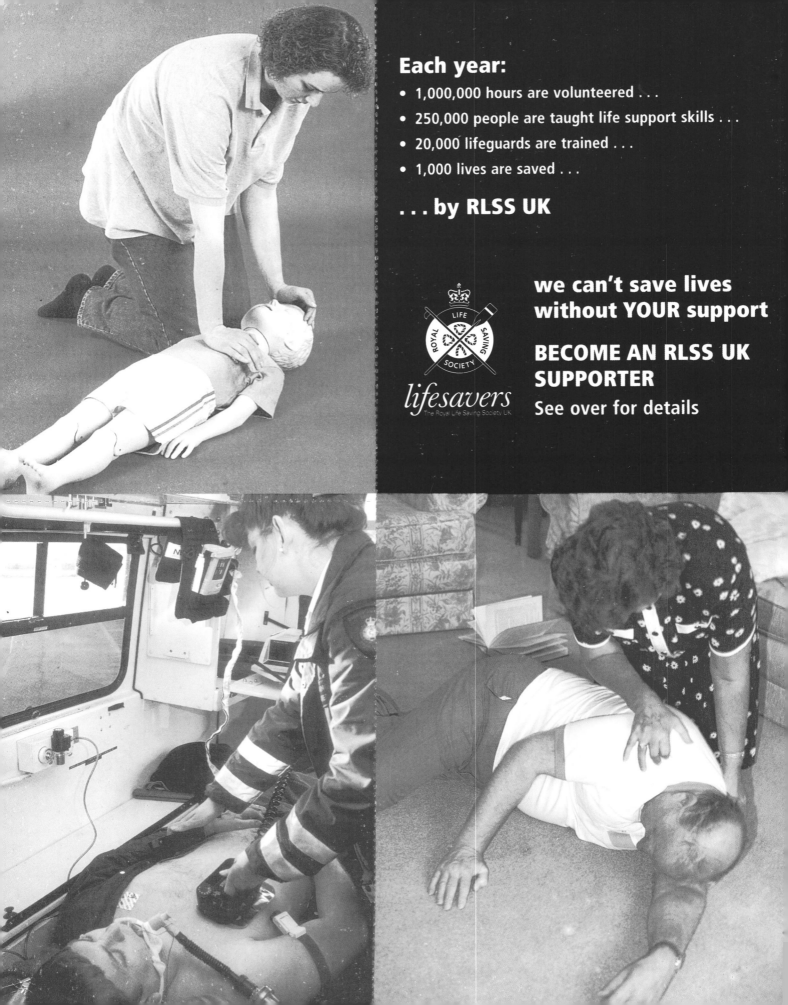

Each year:

- 1,000,000 hours are volunteered . . .
- 250,000 people are taught life support skills . . .
- 20,000 lifeguards are trained . . .
- 1,000 lives are saved . . .

. . . by RLSS UK

lifesavers
The Royal Life Saving Society UK

we can't save lives without YOUR support

BECOME AN RLSS UK SUPPORTER
See over for details